ysm
body bible

Jodie Hedley-Ward is the originator of the *You Sexy Mother* concept and author of the international best-sellers, *You Sexy Mother* and *You Sexy Mother: The Journal.* In demand as a public speaker, Jodie also has a website (www.yousexymother.com.au) which provides inspiration and support to mums around the world. In 2009 she founded the International Motherhood Study alongside Dr Angela Huntsman. Originally from New Zealand, Jodie now lives in Queensland, Australia with her husband David and their two children, Lili and Josh.

Kelli Johnson, who has devised and tested all the training programs in the book, is an international figure champion and now a highly successful personal trainer and member of the IFBB Professional League. Career highlights include winning Miss Australia twice, representing Australia at the world titles and becoming a professional athlete in her 40s. Kelli has a sports science degree and lives in Australia with her husband Colin and daughter Paige. Her website is www.keljohnson.com

What mums are saying about *You Sexy Mother*...

The first time I went on national television and spoke about the *You Sexy Mother* philosophy and 'tired-mum syndrome', an incredible 1600 emails came flooding in within 24 hours. Here is just a snapshot of what you had to say ...

I just wanted to say a great big thank you for your awesome book. I stumbled upon it after talking to my cousin who had found that your words had 'revolutionised' her life. She wouldn't even lend me her copy as she said she often refers to it!

So I went and spent the money and it could not have come at a better time in my life. I am 30 years old and a mother of two beautiful children. I love being at home with them, but I couldn't shake this feeling of discontent and I really felt quite depressed with certain aspects of my life. Mainly how I looked, but also how I had neglected myself so badly that I no longer had any inspiration or goals besides raising these gorgeous kids. When you discussed the 'years of neglect' I almost cried. This was me! It was like you were writing this book just for me!

I want to thank you for inspiring me to get the most out of my life.

Kerry

I discovered your book recently and have to admit my first thought was — why, in this culture, must women be urged to be 'sexy' at all times?

But it wasn't really about the sex, was it! After reading it, I am truly inspired. It dawned on me only a few pages in that this was the most positive take on mothering that I've encountered since joining the 'club'. Almost everything else out there seems to focus on the pain, the tears, the mess and the sleeplessness. Which are all facts of a mother's life ... but dwelling on them indefinitely doesn't help. At first it can be kind of reassuring to read about others suffering a similar 'fate' as a new mother, but after a while, I know that I felt as if I was drowning in a sticky hole, losing hope and pride in my job as a mother, and almost unable to see why anyone would put themselves through it a second time by choice!

Your book has really helped to change my mindset. The job of mothering has been seriously devalued in our culture, but your book will inspire women to reclaim the importance and the joy of that role. I love the sense of positivity with which you've you've approached the topic — without glossing over any of the difficulties.

Thank you for an amazing book!

Robyn

I remember when my daughter was born, I really wished she had come with some kind of instruction manual ... conversations with my husband always used to start with 'I wonder ...' because we really didn't know! I was thinking how amazing it would be if every new mum could have a copy of your book. I wondered if maternity hospitals could give one to each new mum? I am sure it would make a huge difference to how they cope …

I think you are an inspiration and I would love to help you find a way to get your 'Instruction Manual' to mums everywhere!

Sonya

Since I became a mum, my husband and I have drifted further and further apart and I have forgotten to look after myself. About two months ago, something clicked in my head and I thought now is the time to do something about it.

I booked a 10-day detox trip to Bali and then that same night I saw you talking about your book on TV. I purchased the book on the Internet and saved it for my trip. I have only just returned from my trip, which was the best thing I could have done, but what helped me even more was your book. It seemed every section was written just for me.

Narelle

I love that this is more than a one-off, that you're devoting a lot of time, resources and energy into this market, which has been crying out for information, inspiration and a ray of light! We want it all — and there's not much out there that shows us how to get it!

Teresa

My journey so far is that I am a mum of a very spirited, challenging but very affectionate 20-month-old daughter Indiana and she totally turned my world upside down. In addition, we turned our world upside down by relocating, giving up my career and my husband totally changing his. I was at a crossroads a few months ago, just in that limbo land between wanting my old life back and hating myself for not embracing motherhood so passionately as I had my career. I heard about your book on A Current Affair *and went out and bought it. I couldn't put it down and it changed my perspective on so many things. In particular about wanting a life better than the one I had before. Why is it that you only remember the good things about past jobs? I could only remember the travel, the money, people I had met and conveniently forgot the long hours, the deadlines, the pressure and the lack of time for the people that matter the most to me. I didn't know who I was outside of my job and it was totally out of my control.*

It is so refreshing to have this book remind us that it is okay to think about you and, in fact, if you do, the rest will just naturally follow. I am sure you have received many, many other emails just like this one. I have already recommended your book to many of my friends.

Raelene

I took it home in my pile with me last night to read and I couldn't stop reading. From the moment I started reading the introduction 'If tired was not an option' and the way you described that 'aha' moment of no longer being constrained by being busy, or tired, or those tags we all use — it struck a chord — I'm sick of saying that I'm busy, everyone is, we need a new state of being and your attitude and fired-up drive to change your self-image was very inspiring!

Tee

Just writing to say thank you for your book. I have made my vision board and it is on display in the dining area. I watch the light dance off it every day as I move towards my authentic self/life and start to build bridges to where I would like to be. My board started off small and it increased in size as I added words, poems and special sayings kept over the years.

Catherine

I just wanted to let you know that I bought your book this afternoon. It's like your book jumped off the shelf at me. I can't even begin to tell you how much I need this book and so far your words have struck such a chord with me. My journey is now beginning as I read your book and I am finding it inspirational and life-changing already.

After skimming through your book in the store I decided I would actually slow down and order myself something really nice for lunch. So, I sat in a nice coffee shop reading your book, enjoying a fabulous lunch, and for the first time in two years felt no guilt about having time away. It was a revelation! And, afterwards, on my way back to the car, I actually entered a lingerie shop for the first time in many years and decided that as soon as I finish breastfeeding, I am going to buy myself some beautiful underwear as a reward to myself for feeding two children!

Jodee

The book has taken me through a journey of self-assurance; my babies are 20 & 17! Our son went off to university this year and what a heart-wrenching time, so I've read your book, got out the old photo albums and family videos and had a wonderful time remembering being a new mum. I would do some things differently — but not many!

Thanks for sharing and highlighting how wonderful it is having littlies — this has helped heal some of the heartache.

Helen

It is amazing that I actually bought your book and let it sit in my room for about three months before I felt the time was right for me to read it — I had to be ready to take it on. I want to thank you so much — I just wish I could hire you out to come and do some one-on-one sessions with me!

Scherone

ysm
body bible

JODIE HEDLEY-WARD

WITH KELLI JOHNSON

Foreword by Terri Irwin

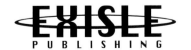

EXISLE
PUBLISHING

First published 2010

Exisle Publishing Limited,
'Moonrising', Narone Creek Road, Wollombi, NSW 2325, Australia.
P.O. Box 60-490, Titirangi, Auckland 0642, New Zealand.
www.exislepublishing.com

National Library of Australia Cataloguing-in-Publication entry

Hedley-Ward, Jodie, 1976- .
You sexy mother body bible / Jodie Hedley-Ward with Kelli Johnson.
1st ed.
9781921497827 (pbk.)
Includes bibliographical references.
Self-actualization (Psychology) in women.
Physical fitness for women
Women—Health and hygiene.
Women—Nutrition.
Dewey Number: 613.7045

ISBN 978-1-921497-82-7

10 9 8 7 6 5 4 3 2 1

Text and cover design by Christabella Designs
Photography by Dallas Olsen
Printed in Singapore by KHL Printing Co.Pte.Ltd

This book uses paper sourced under ISO 14001 guidelines from well-managed forests and other controlled sources.

Dedicated to every woman who finds her way to this book …

May you find within these pages the answers you seek to questions
you possibly haven't even been able to voice yet.

Contents

Foreword

When it comes to coaching someone to a place of total health and fitness, nobody does it better than Kelli.

I was first introduced to Kelli a couple of years ago when Steve's sister Joy and her husband, Frank, started their weight training. I was especially impressed with Kelli's achievements as she is only three years younger than me and is competing at the top in her body-shaping events. She is an exceptional athlete who only wants to help others reach their personal best.

I have been nothing short of astounded by the results I have experienced after following Kelli's nutrition and exercise plan. Since I am very involved with hands-on wildlife work, the strength I have gained by eating right and getting fit has really helped when it comes to our crocodile research. Especially when I have to hang on to a 4-metre-long dinosaur!

I have also found that Kelli's routine has led to better sleeping, clear thinking, and the ability to cope with life's stresses. The other bonus of getting into shape is the confidence in attending red-carpet events and knowing that I can promote a healthy body instead of an incredibly skinny one!

Best of all, I've gained a great friend. Thanks Kelli!

TERRI IRWIN
Australia Zoo

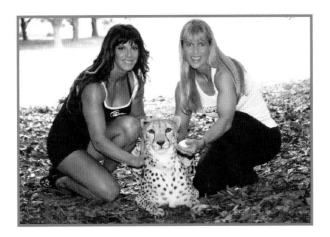

Thanks to ...

Each of the following people has sprinkled a little of their own unique magic upon this project and I am so grateful for their contributions and support.

Kelli Johnson and Terri Irwin

Mary O'Dwyer, Dr Angela Huntsman and Anders Lindgreen

Lorna Jane – for providing the clothing featured throughout the book

Dallas Olsen and Antoinette Wilkins for their respective photographic and styling expertise

The amazing team at Exisle Publishing

Annah Stretton, Donna and Gerry Morris and Deborah Parker for their ongoing support

My wonderful husband David, and finally ...

To Lili and Josh – tell me again, how did I get to be the luckiest mum in the world?

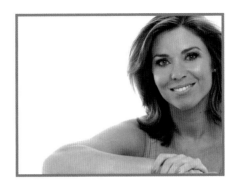

Your Best Body Yet

'24 months to a new body!'

Let me ask you a question — how likely are you to purchase a magazine with the above tagline, as opposed to one that reads 'Lose 20 kg in four weeks'? I'll tell you right now — not very likely at all.

The truth is, sculpting an athletic body takes time and effort, depending on what condition you wish it to be in and what condition you were in when you started. It has to be earned, but this is also what makes it so rewarding. Your body becomes your very own Oscar statue; something that money cannot buy and that no one can ever take away from you. It becomes a source of great confidence and, unlike a trophy, it is very useful and will enable you to get ahead in life and create some well-deserved momentum. And even if you won't achieve your desired end result tomorrow, it will gradually build — every small success will make the journey easier and that smile on your face a little wider.

The program that follows has been designed with you in mind — a busy, multifaceted woman, whose body has undergone a major transition as a result of giving birth. It is real, it is honest, and it works. Be kind to yourself as you approach this wonderful turning point in your life, knowing that time and effort can take you anywhere you want to go — but you must allow enough of both if you ever hope to reach the end goal.

Be easy about it all and enjoy the ride!

Go confidently in the direction of your dreams. Live the life you have imagined.
HENRY DAVID THOREAU

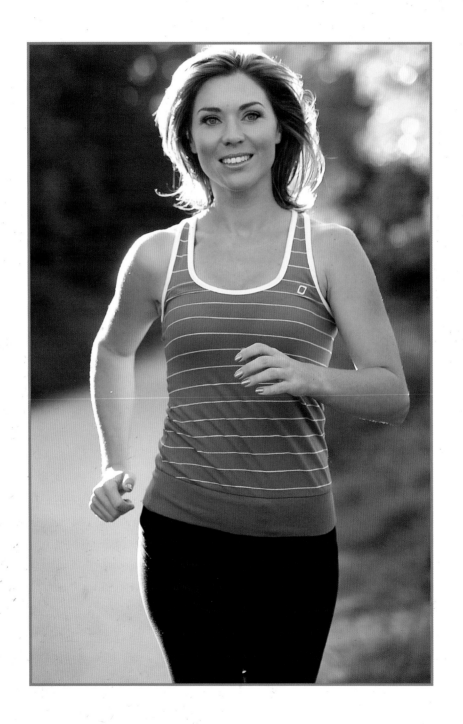

Flab to Fab in *Just* 12 Weeks!

Jodie's 12-week challenge

Our deepest fear is not that we are inadequate. Our deepest fear is that we are powerful
beyond measure. It is our light, not our darkness that most frightens us.
We ask ourselves, Who am I to be brilliant, gorgeous, talented, fabulous?
Actually, who are you not to be?

MARIANNE WILLIAMSON

In the next section you can read what happened when I met acclaimed health and fitness trainer Kelli Johnson, and began a 12-week intensive program designed to change the way I approached nutrition and exercise forever. I will share every aspect of that journey, the highs and the inevitable challenges ... and ultimately the wonderful long-term changes that I have enjoyed ever since.

My goal in working with Kelli was to use myself as a human guinea pig – to test out Kelli's strategies and tools and see if they could *really* work for a normal mum like me. I wanted to help other mums avoid wasting precious time and money and instead hop on the fast-track to guaranteed success ...

It is important for you to know that Kelli trained me and gave so generously of her time and extensive knowledge during this period and she did so for free. I didn't even discuss the details of writing a book with her initially. I just asked her if she would be willing to work with me towards creating something powerful for mums that could change their relationships with their bodies forever, and without any need for further convincing she said 'YES!'

The very next day, we were on our way ... Nobody was more surprised than me at the speed of all this. I now know that Kelli is not one for sitting around and talking about results — she just gets on with it and creates them.

I wanted to make sure I worked with someone who would invest the time and energy in this collaboration because they genuinely wanted to help other mums ... not because of the money. That was my litmus test if you like, and Kelli passed with flying colours.

She, like me, really just wants to help you. It's that simple! So join me now as I share the first tentative (and at times scary) steps towards my new reality.

My journey begins ...

Have you ever wanted to experience something but realised that what you wanted was so far removed from your reality that you didn't even know how to articulate it? That's how I felt at this point. I knew precisely what my body wasn't, and I had become very good at camouflaging parts of it that I wanted to hide and emphasising my better aspects.

In a former life I had been very involved in the design and marketing of plus-size women's fashion in the UK — conducting focus-group research with plus-size women and working alongside the design team to help translate the women's desire to look and feel beautiful into clothes that made them feel great. Although I had never been plus-size myself, I had learnt all the tricks of concealing and revealing in all the right places — to the point where I had begun to use that skill as a reason to avoid getting up a sweat at my local gym!

Good is the enemy of great.
JIM COLLINS

The saying 'Good is the enemy of great' (from the wonderful book by Jim Collins, titled *Good to Great*) certainly applies to matters of health and fitness. Although I was *okay* in terms of my physical size and my ability to run and jump about – I wasn't feeling *great*. As my life became busier (who would have thought that becoming an author would be so hectic?) I started abusing coffee to the point where I would reach for a caffeine fix to give me the energy I needed to keep going at the pace I wanted. I would wake up feeling sluggish, and at times feel as if a bulldozer had run over me. 'Nothing a coffee can't fix,' I would say, and I would continue to rely on my positive attitude and my faithful friend coffee to get me through another day.

I probably would have continued that way feeling pretty average about my body shape and energy levels and believing that walking around with a cloudy head and foggy thoughts was 'normal' if it hadn't been for a rather gorgeous little boy called Josh, who at just two years of age received an important health diagnosis following an extended period of being very poorly. My son's diagnosis of coeliac disease sent my world into a spin and resulted in my embarking on a search for 'optimal health', something I wasn't sure I had ever truly experienced.

If you have ever seen a person completely transform their health, and alongside that, their personality, you will understand how incredibly inspirational it is to those around them. Josh had reached such a low level of health prior to his diagnosis, with a distended stomach and unexplained weight loss. He had all but given up eating food except for dry crackers and the occasional apple slice. He was chronically lethargic and clung to his mum like a koala bear to a tree – offering delicious cuddles that were soured by the worry I felt at every moment regarding his health.

By eliminating wheat and gluten from his diet, within a matter of weeks Josh was like a different kid. His energy levels were soaring, he was putting on weight and his stomach was slowly returning to its normal size. Most fascinating, however, was the fact that his moods had improved beyond all recognition. Gone were the severe mood swings that seemed to accompany his deteriorating health, replaced by a happy, giggly boy who delighted in simple games and pulling funny faces once again.

I began to play around with the notion that if Josh's moods and energy levels could be transformed so radically, could it be possible to do the same for an adult? A homeopath I had been visiting with Josh planted the seed in my mind for the idea of pursuing *optimal health*.

'But I think I *am* pretty healthy,' I said to him one day, to which he replied, 'What if you don't even know what good health feels like? What if you thought you were okay simply because you had never actually experienced optimal health before?'

I started to see how relative this whole notion of health really is. Healthy relative to what? Fit relative to what? We are all coming from different starting points and with completely different conditioning in terms of what we think constitutes good health based on our unique family history and the influences of those around us.

I decided that optimal health was something I wanted to achieve, and Josh was to be my biggest inspiration — I had never before seen someone's health transform so radically before my very eyes. It changed my belief about what was possible and allowed me to open up to the idea of achieving a state of optimal rather than just mediocre health.

All I needed was the right person to help me. How hard could that be?

Finding Kelli

It's one thing to *want* a great body and another thing to *get* one. I had spent years of my life on and off searching for the elusive 'solution' or trainer that would make my goal of a fit, toned, strong body a reality. Some trainers had given me results while I was focused on working with them, but nothing had morphed into the kind of lifestyle solution that I was looking for — something that was fun, addictive and easy to follow for the rest of my life.

A critical moment for me came about after a less than enjoyable dental experience when I ended up being seen by a junior dentist as the principal dentist to whom I had been recommended was no longer taking new patients. I made a decision that I believe led to my eventually finding Kelli Johnson. I know it seems a rather large leap, but stay with me because this point is very important. In fact it was a major defining moment in my life.

I was so mad that I had allowed myself to go from requesting the 'best dentist around' to accepting what I thought was mediocre treatment (at best) from someone much less experienced. So from that day onwards I declared that I would never allow myself to accept anything less than the best when it came to professionals, mentors or people assisting me in life in some way.

A couple of days later as I was pondering the idea of getting myself off to the gym

with the gym-junkie gene, shall we say — so I did not have the luxury of learning what I know now at a young age!

Many women of our parents' generation were brought up to believe that we should just accept the body that motherhood gives us (yes, pelvic floor dysfunction and all!) and essentially ride out the remainder of our journey here on planet Earth in a less than optimal physical vehicle. I never really accepted this theory and always rebelled against the idea that my best body (and life) ought to be the one I had prior to becoming a mum!

I walked into Kelli's home gym today with a size-12 body that looked pretty okay in clothes, but I was not surprised when Kelli described me as being 'skinny-fat'. If you have never come across the term before, it offers an accurate description of people like me who although not 'large', are not actually toned and fit. It's one thing to look good in your clothes, but quite another to have the kind of toned, tight body that looks great in a swimsuit. I feel reasonably confident about my body but for a long time I have wanted to experience a level of strength, fitness and energy that up until now has eluded me.

As a writer and researcher, I invariably spend a lot of time at the computer or sitting in meetings. My life, by the very nature of my work, is relatively sedentary. I do try to get out and run around with the kids as much as I can but it is not consistent enough to create the kind of improvement I am looking for. I am excited at a personal level about what working with Kelli will achieve for me in a physical sense, but more importantly I am excited to see how the strategies I employ to get there will be able to work for mothers everywhere. In this way, I can let go of my past conditioning, and state with conviction that your best body is possible at any time in your life. I fully intend to have a better body at the end of this journey than I did at 25 or 30. I am more conscious now of my lifestyle choices and how they impact on my energy levels and general well-being. I am probably more motivated to look and feel great too as I now have kids and a husband who rely on me to be at my best. By letting myself down, I am inadvertently affecting those I love also. How motivating is that!

Another rather confronting aspect of my first training session with Kelli was the full-length mirror that runs down one side of her home gym. I admitted to Kelli that there aren't any full-length mirrors in my house and I am not used to looking at my body as honestly as this. I had also not weighed myself for years, and even stepping up on the scales felt scary. I also admitted to Kelli that I have carried this image of myself around as being 'a natural, low-maintenance kinda girl' for so long that it was acting as a cop-out and preventing me from creating the kind of fit, strong and toned body I secretly longed for. I had wrongly associated being fit and healthy with being obsessive and vain ... Meeting someone like Kelli was just the motivation I needed to reassess my attitude to fitness and shake up those erroneous stereotypes that had done nothing but keep me in a holding pattern and distanced me from the happiness and joy I was truly seeking. Talk about self-sabotaging behaviour!

The other important issue that came up for me today was the idea that as mums we can often accept second-best, or settle for less than we truly want and deserve. Kelli charges the same as many other trainers in my local area, yet most of them have never competed at a national or international level and do not have her proven track record in getting results for clients.

I have finally come to the realisation that the difference between paying for the best person in their field to teach and guide you, versus a very average person, is usually relatively small. The difference in the results you will see in your life, however, is major. We need to demand the best for ourselves and seek out the best coaches, support people and mentors we can find. There is always a way to get what you want, and even teaming up with one or more friends in order to pay for the expertise of the best trainer you can find is going to get you a far better result than doing nothing or shopping around on your own for the cheapest option.

Kelli also said that most people believe they need to be mega-fit already before they can train with her, and many are embarrassed to ask if she would train them because they don't think they are 'good enough' or 'slim enough' to work with her. I guess it goes back to what one of my favourite holistic health authors, Louise Hay, writes, that most of us do not think we are *good enough* or *worthy enough*, and that is what holds us back in life.

I am working with Kelli for one hour every Tuesday, but because of her passion around creating transformations for her clients, she will be emailing me nutrition and exercise plans for the week so that I feel supported every step of the way. I feel like I am heading to a place I have never been before. I was not the sporty girl at school but rather the 'good student', so I know that whatever I can achieve, you can achieve. I am starting from a place of relative ignorance — I feel strongly that this is the start of something very profound for me, and I am sure that by achieving my health and fitness goals I will create the self-confidence and momentum I am looking for, to go on and achieve phenomenal results in every other area of my life.

Stay tuned!

Week 1 — a newfound clarity

After being warned by Kelli that I might feel a little out of sorts or foggy during the initial five-day detox program, I was pleasantly surprised when after just two days of eating 'clean' my head felt clearer than it had for many years. I was waking up feeling sharp and ready to jump out of bed, and I loved the contrast with my former reality where it would take a shower and a plunger of coffee to get me fully into gear in the mornings.

I was changing from a very sporadic, haphazard eating pattern to a very structured routine and my body seemed to be loving it. Kelli explained that our bodies love rhythm and routine. They like to know that food is coming on a regular timetable, and that way they don't feel a need to store food as fat in case of a potential famine in the future. Kelli had me eating every three hours from the time I got up, and the hardest thing for me at first was actually eating the amount of food on my program. I wasn't used to eating so regularly, and I started to realise that perhaps I hadn't been eating *enough* food up until now. There were times when I would have breakfast and then nothing but a coffee and a chocolate biscuit until well into the afternoon — no wonder my energy levels had been failing me.

Could it be true that I hadn't in fact been eating enough? How many other mums, I wondered, were eating too little (and probably the wrong stuff) and wondering why they didn't have the energy (or the body) they wanted?

'Energy gets energy,' Kelli told me, and I repeated that like a silent mantra all week. 'If you want energy, you've got to exercise to get it. It doesn't work the other way round. Don't wait for the energy to come before you start exercising, it just won't happen and you'll end up sabotaging your chances of health and vitality forever.'

'Muscles need to be fed,' Kelli instructed, and so I had to adapt to incorporating a little protein into most of my six meals throughout the day. This proved to be a bit challenging at first as I was used to reaching for a chocolate biscuit or a piece of fruit with my morning cuppa — so the thought of having rice cakes with cottage cheese and sliced chicken breast just seemed odd! I persevered, however, and loved the feeling of being full and the energy that came from eating something substantial like that early in the day.

To say the transformation in my energy levels that week was remarkable is an understatement. By the end of the first week I was turning to my husband and saying incredulously, 'I don't even feel like I need a coffee today!' Which for me at that point was amazing. Both Kelli and my naturopath had expressed a desire to get me to a place where I could drink coffee because I enjoyed it, not because I needed it.

Whether your crutch is coffee, Coke, sugary foods or salty crackers, lots of us rely on unhealthy pick-me-ups to get us through the day. I wanted to learn the strategies to enjoy a full, fun life without that crutch, and I saw very early on that this wasn't just a real possibility — it was something that I could achieve very quickly.

The biggest challenge for me lay in the training side of the equation. I already had a gym membership that up until now had been doing very little except collecting dust. I now found that getting to the gym to run on the treadmill was one thing, but committing to a 30-minute weight-training session three times a week was proving to be my biggest challenge.

I reached the end of the first week and had to congratulate myself on my dietary changes and the soaring energy levels I had experienced. I was honest with Kelli and told her that the weight-training had held me back, although I had managed to fit in three additional cardio sessions since we last met. She agreed that this was a 'process', and praised me for not beating myself up over the weight-training and instead focusing on the positive changes I had made regarding my eating.

And with that little boost and a wonderful feeling of 'I can do this!' rising up inside me, I concluded the first week on a total high.

Maybe, just maybe, I can actually do this, I thought as my head hit the pillow on the last night!

Finding my way

The next few weeks proved difficult. I was so unprepared and it seemed like I was just wading through sticky jam trying to follow Kelli's nutritional plan. I found myself out at a café with no snacks in my bag, starving because I had been at the gym at 6am, and with no 'good' choices staring at me from the food counter ... what's a girl to do?

'Get organised!' Kelli declared defiantly when I asked her how I could possibly stick to the plan when my life was so busy. She'd heard it all before! She reminded me, without so much as a hint of superiority, that she too was a mum and that she had made it to the top of her game with a small baby in tow, whilst being a single mother trying to study and make ends meet. That sure gave me some food for thought! But *how* exactly did she do it? It seemed to me that fitting in the exercise wasn't proving nearly as hard as actually eating the right things up to six times a day.

'You have to get organised the night before,' Kelli reminded me. 'Don't expect to wake up from a deep sleep with a strong desire to train and eat well without putting in the preparation required.' I could understand this because I advocate a bit of night-time preparation in *You Sexy Mother*, to ensure a smooth (or at least smoother) transition into the day. I started to think ahead and while making dinner I would get out a container for my salad the next day, and begin putting bits and pieces into it as I ferreted about in the fridge. It didn't matter whether I was eating at home or not the next day; I soon worked out that if I had a healthy salad ready and waiting for me in the fridge or in my bag, the chances of eating 'clean and green' were always high. If I relied on the fact that I would be home the next day and then went out unexpectedly without taking food with me, it was a recipe for disaster.

Not exactly rocket science, you might say, but the simple strategy of getting myself to focus the night before on what kind of day I wanted to have really started to make a huge difference. If I was training the next morning, then my water bottle would be filled, my iPod charged up and clothes laid out by my bed so they would be the first things I would see upon rising. The less time I allowed for those voices in my head to take hold, the better. I was determined to follow Kelli's success strategies and felt confident that if she could do it as a mum, so could I.

I had a few more trips to the supermarket than normal as I realised I was eating a lot more fruit and vegetables than before. I also realised that it had been over a week since I last slipped a chocolate biscuit into my mouth and I hadn't even missed it. My habit of raising my energy levels via sugar and caffeine had been replaced by a daily struggle to keep up with the relentless nature of my new eating plan. The only thing I had complained about was having to stop so many times during the day to eat — not a bad problem to have, I guess.

When someone asked me if I was on a special diet, as I tucked into a banana and chocolate protein shake at the kids' swimming lessons one morning, I had to laugh. The old-fashioned diet concept was so far removed from what I was now experiencing. I was starting to consider myself more as an expensive luxury car — requiring premium fuel to keep me running at optimal speed. As I looked around me and saw a sea of muffins, cakes and coffees, I realised exactly why Kelli's nutrition plan works. It focuses on *fuelling* the body rather than drip-feeding it with the traditional high-sugar snacks we mums can easily learn to exist on if we don't start becoming more mindful of our nutrition.

The world becomes my mirror

The results started to happen, and week by week muscles started to reveal themselves in places that I had never seen before. To say I was surprised is an understatement. Although I had never been a particularly big person, muscle and tone had not played a large part in my experience up until now. What was interesting is that I was learning to be prepared for the changes in my body and shape, but I was totally unprepared for the reactions from those around me.

I observed the comments and the looks the way an author observes all life around them — in a pretty detached way. I would visit Kelli once a week and share what was happening, thinking she would be shocked. Instead she just laughed and told me about a time when she had walked into a fruit and vegetable store, past a young couple, and overheard the guy say 'Now I'm feeling intimidated!' Kelli said she hadn't really thought much about how others reacted to her up until that point. It had made her take a closer look at her body and wonder if she really looked that different from most women. The sad fact is that our society is becoming so predominantly overweight that anyone who challenges that status quo becomes a target for those who are less than comfortable in their own skins.

I was nowhere near the physique Kelli was in the above example, but I was noticing within my own social circle, at the kids' activities where I would show up each week looking progressively leaner, more toned and eating differently, that it challenged many women around me. It was as if my decision to change my physical reality made them feel uncomfortable about staying where they were. Some were complimentary and some were downright rude, choosing to comment more on my new food choices than my improved energy levels or toned body. I started to see that many of them put words in my mouth, trying to get me to tell a story of struggle and deprivation: 'You aren't eating good food any more, are you?' or 'Are you still doing that diet thing?' No matter how many times I tried to correct them and say I wasn't on any diet but merely choosing healthier options, they didn't want to hear it.

I quickly realised the futility of that game and decided to just carry on with my plan regardless — I knew from experience that their comments weren't even about me, they were always about what was going on inside for them. So the first few weeks were dramatic in terms of my results, but I also felt relatively isolated in some ways as I was still trying to integrate my new strategies into my life and politely navigate the social obligations of accepting sweet treats at every turn and refusing invitations that would impact on my commitment to eat well and work out each week.

To say I was pleased I did was an understatement because what came next really shook things up in a good way ...

Results ripple out!

Jodie walked into our office one day looking toned and confident, with these amazing arm muscles. I just looked at her and said, 'Wow ... whatever you are doing, I want to do it too!'
LISA LINDLEY, PSYCHOLOGIST AND FRIEND

The first time that the way I was feeling on the inside was accurately reflected back to me by the outside world was when I went to drop off some copies of *You Sexy Mother* to a good friend of mine who runs an amazing post-natal depression support group on Australia's Sunshine Coast. Lisa had known me for about a year, after attending a

You Sexy Mother event and contacting me to ask if I would speak to her group. We had developed a wonderful friendship based upon our shared passion for helping women feel good and doing whatever it takes to support them on that journey.

When I walked in after not having seen Lisa for a couple of months, she stopped in her tracks, cupped her hands to her mouth and exclaimed, 'What have you been doing? You look fantastic!' Beyond the ego boost, what I felt was a kind of validation that the changes I was experiencing internally in terms of my renewed energy, improved sleep and clear thinking were now extending to a tangible physical improvement that was inspiring change in others. 'Whatever you are doing, I want to do it too!' she continued. Now, instead of making those around me uncomfortable, a sort of change started to take place whereby my results were inspiring others to make positive changes too.

The next time I walked into Lisa's workplace, two mums who worked there told me they were now training with Kelli as a result of seeing the changes in me. That was cool. Very cool! My guinea-pig experiment was working faster than I could ever have imagined. Without my having to say anything, everywhere I went I would get people asking me what I did to stay in shape and have so much energy.

I began to notice all around me the women who 'got it' versus the women who truly didn't. One group seemed to be radiating joy and managing to laugh at the silly things that make up your day as a mum. The others, by contrast, were spending a large chunk of time lamenting the fact that they felt overwhelmed or frustrated with their lives and children. I was beginning to see that the people they felt most frustrated with were themselves, and their sense of being overwhelmed by everything had more to do with the fact that they were talking about it rather than getting on and doing something to change it.

It wasn't just women who were affected by the changes in me; my own husband was so inspired by my commitment to this new way of life that one day he just sat me down and said, 'I want to do everything that you're doing — eat the way you're eating and train alongside you.' That was a huge bonus as it meant that I was only having to prepare one meal in the evenings and could buy the same food for both of us. We even started inspiring more healthy choices in our kids as they saw us prepare gourmet salads and delicious-looking fruit salads that often ended up having two little people devouring most of them.

Bumps in the road

As with any journey, the highs were peppered with lows and moments where I felt it was all just too hard. At one point I fell sick and couldn't eat anything – I just felt rotten. My old thought patterns emerged and I started finding myself thinking that maybe this new, healthy eating routine was the cause, and perhaps I should just go back to eating more of the comfort food my body seemed to enjoy before. I emailed Kelli to cancel one of our training sessions and told her I was on the sofa feeling sorry for myself, and I asked her if she had any advice. It seemed like the response took less than a minute – Kelli knew that emotionally I was in trouble and there was no time to lose.

She said that no matter what, it was imperative that I stay really hydrated and rest. She said some olive leaf extract (which I had already been taking on the recommendation of my naturopath) would be good for my general immune system, along with a good dose of vitamin C. She almost seemed to read my mind, and said that coming down with a cold or flu is sometimes just part of life and that it probably would have happened no matter what – so 'don't blame your healthy new routine!'

This was just the jolt I needed to make me realise how clever our minds can be at sabotaging our success. Here I was feeling so incredibly good about my body, my energy levels and my commitment to a healthy, active lifestyle, then one little cold comes along and immediately I am debating internally about whether or not I should carry on or go back to my old ways!

Luckily within a couple of days I was completely restored – I couldn't believe it. I had gone from feeling as low as I could possibly imagine to feeling 100% back to full strength and vitality ... I'd never known anything like it. With my energy restored, so too was my ability to think clearly and make sound judgements. I slowly began working out again, and at my next week's training session with Kelli I shared my emotional journey from the past week. Kelli wasn't at all surprised when I told her how I had started questioning everything and wondering if it was all just too hard. She said she sees it all the time with new clients – the ones who work through it and continue the journey are the ones who realise life will always present us with obstacles and barriers to achieving our desired goals. We just need to see them as inevitable bumps in the road, not mountains that are impossible to climb. She reminded me that I had crossed over a very significant threshold by choosing to quickly re-establish my healthy lifestyle and not dwell on the sickness.

From that point on, I noticed the voices in my head seemed quieter and less persistent when it came to the small challenges along the way. Kelli was right. There were many social events and dinner invitations that presented nutritional challenges to me on a regular basis, but I just saw them for what they were and worked at making the best choice in each moment, focusing on one day at a time.

Redefining me

It's hard to pinpoint exactly when it happened, but at some stage on this journey I was no longer thinking of myself in the same way as before. I was actually starting to see myself as one of the 'fit' crowd — someone who *belonged* in the gym, rather than the girl in the baggy tee-shirt trying to pretend she knew how to use that strange elliptical machine in the corner. I mean, how intimidating is *that* to a new gym member — legs going up and down, arms backwards and forwards … it took a month before I plucked up the courage to ask how to use that machine!

I think the change in my own self-perception came about partly as a result of physical changes (dropping a dress size or two and seeing thigh muscles where before there were none sure helps) but more importantly from the reflection of myself in others' eyes. People were asking my advice about what gym they should join or where to get good workout clothes — simple questions, but strangely, not ones that I had ever really been asked before. The 'fit' mums were seeking me out, so it seemed. They were making a concerted effort to talk to me in the school playground or at the park, as if I now probably had more in common with them than before. I can't even explain it (as I'm pretty much the kind of person who will talk to anyone if they so much as smile at me). All I know is that my life was changing in inexplicable ways and people were holding me up as an expert in something that was still very new to me, still a work in progress. It took many more months before my self-confidence and internal view of myself matched up to the fit person others were seeing externally.

At first I just thought Jodie was on a 'health kick' — she would turn up to the kids' swimming lessons with her fruit, nuts and healthy goodies while the rest of us devoured our muffins and coffees from the café. I thought it wouldn't last and would be a passing phase like with most mums, but Jodie really surprised us all. She started to look amazing and she had more energy than the rest of us put together! That's when we started asking her what her secret way was — we wanted to look and feel like that too!

MEGAN, MUM OF TWO

We all know that you can change your physical appearance pretty quickly (cosmetic surgery is a clear example of this) but it will take much longer for you to internalise those changes. This is what we call body dysmorphia, and it is the reason why anorexia and bulimia are two of the hardest mental disorders to treat — the person's external appearance does not match how they feel about themselves on the inside, and it can be very challenging for health professionals and mental health workers to overcome that inconsistency.

Luckily for me, the period of time when I experienced feelings of body dysmorphia did not last long as I started to really connect internally with this fit and healthy person people were responding to as I went about my day.

This was a wonderfully integrated and fully connected place to arrive at — mind, body and soul. Better than any expensive gift, retail therapy or compliment, it was authentic, hard won and under my control. Unlike diets or short bursts at the gym that in the past had created a degree of success, I felt as if I had finally learned the rules of the game. I had the knowledge and the experience to carry this forward in my life indefinitely, and I knew that if I relaxed a little or even went off my program for a while, I had everything I needed to plug back in at any moment and get myself right back to a place of total health and self-love any time I wanted. It was liberating beyond belief.

I found myself being overwhelmed by a sense of 'Why hasn't anyone taught me this stuff before?' I wish I had known how to eat and exercise correctly during high school as it would have saved me from so much destructive behaviour in the form of dieting and emotional self-abuse. I had dabbled with dieting and pushing things too far at a relatively early age and then thankfully come through it quite young. By the time I was at university I was a very vocal campaigner for women looking and feeling gorgeous regardless of their size, and I always felt very body-confident despite being much larger than I am now.

I celebrated my curves and went on to study and work with plus-size women. This passion of mine continued when I landed a dream job in the UK, working for an Italian women's fashion company who were in the process of launching a plus-size mail-order catalogue and needed someone with my specialised knowledge to help make it a success. I had the time of my life, facilitating focus groups throughout England with plus-size women, where they would share openly how it felt to walk into a store and not be able to find anything that would fit, let alone make them look fantastic. The sadness, grief, anger and shame that these amazing women shared touched me deeply and made me more committed to doing things in my life to empower women to feel great in their skins.

I also had the pleasure of overseeing photo shoots in London with some of the world's leading plus-size models. These women were gorgeous – inside and out. They realised that they were positive role models for young girls and they really believed they were making a difference within the magazines that would feature them.

All of these events from my past and the faces of these amazing women I had spoken to over the years came flooding back to me as I sat contemplating the newfound knowledge I had since meeting Kelli. Not all of us are lucky enough to be raised by people who understand the simple principles involved in looking and feeling good in our own skins, and some of us have a much longer and more challenging journey to get to a good place. I just knew that I had to write a book with Kelli and share her knowledge so that we could help speed things up for those mums who were ready to listen. If we could help just one mum connect the dots a little faster and make positive leaps forward in terms of feeling good in her own skin, then it would be fantastic.

This book is powerful and simple. If you read it and take action, you will be rewarded with the kind of body you can love. It won't be a perfect body (as without airbrushing there really is no such thing) but it will be the best body you can own, and how many of us can honestly say we are currently living inside that? Believe that this is possible and allow yourself enough time to see if my words are true before you dismiss them. I have done the work and followed the plan – I know it works. So from that position of total knowing, I fully expect that you will enjoy success and transformation beyond your wildest dreams too.

Go create and enjoy – create a new life and enjoy the body that comes from being active and dedicated to a life of well-being!

Doing it to living it ...

The program becomes a vital, wonderful part of my daily life

I wanted to share with you the transition from working hard at 'doing' the program to effortlessly merging the 'rules' I learnt into my daily life which, like yours, can be pretty busy at times. For me life revolves around trying to fit publishing deadlines, research meetings, speaking engagements and media interviews in and around the weekly busyness of our family routine – for you it might be juggling work outside the home with your family schedule, or balancing all the different (and at times conflicting) needs when you have a baby and older children in the household. It doesn't matter what we do as mothers, we all tend to extend ourselves to the limit at times.

I found that I started to use whatever time I had available to do something, rather than pushing myself to fit in a full one-hour workout on a specific number of days per week. That means I am more flexible with what activity I do each day, and I mix it up depending on where I am and what crops up. If my husband needs to get to work particularly early and I can't get to the gym as planned, I will just pop on my running shoes and go for a quick run around the block, followed by some walking lunges up and down my driveway and a stretch. This might be 30 minutes all up but I know it's enough to make a difference, and I know that a little bit of something most days is far more effective than a perfect one-hour cardio and resistance training session at my local gym once a week or month.

I spent the first 12 weeks with Kelli really studying her principles – both the exercise and nutrition guidelines and the strategies for integrating them into my life. Now I can have fun playing around with that knowledge. I don't have to follow any specific nutrition plan now; I simply choose from the meal and snack options that I know work best for my body and, within reason, if I stick to that 80% of the time, my weight and body will continue to look and feel its best. You can't get there straight away, you have to feel your way into it and follow things a little more strictly at first in order to learn the tools that will work for you over the long term. But once you arrive at that point, it's great to know you can eat out, take it easier whilst on holiday and even do what you like 20% of the time without worry ... it just starts to get easier and easier. Your body adopts a new set point in terms of weight and you can settle into a nice routine that suits your personality.

So if you love meeting up with friends on a Sunday morning for a delicious brunch at the local café, you can still do that. If you like to completely rest at the weekend and not even look at your trainers, you can do that too ... just so long as when Monday rolls around you get back into it and get your body moving again.

There are no hard and fast rules to all of this; it is designed to work in real life, and to be something you can sustain in the long term. The reality for most people, however, is that for a couple of months you are going to need to focus more intensely on making it happen, otherwise you won't achieve the kinds of results that will motivate you to stick to this new, healthy way of life.

How far can you go?
The IFBB Queensland Figure Championships

This journey started for me because of one woman by the name of Vickie. You can read all about her personal journey in the case study on page 115. During my 12-week challenge with Kelli, Vickie was training at a very high level for the Queensland IFBB Figure Championships. On the day of the big event, I went along to support Vickie and see exactly how far her training with Kelli had taken her. Kelli was a judge at the event, and there was a guest appearance by Terri Irwin and her daughter Bindi who jumped up on stage to share their passion for a healthy, fit lifestyle.

I was so inspired by Terri's message to the women at the event. She said that the training with Kelli and her focus on nutrition were what enabled her to cope with the incredible demands of her busy lifestyle — running an iconic, internationally successful wildlife attraction alongside her dedication as a mum and wildlife conservationist. She urged all women (especially mums) to get up and get active, so they too would have all the energy and self-confidence required to pursue an extraordinary life. Bindi reinforced Terri's empowering words by saying that she had been so inspired by her mum's healthy approach to life that she too was committed to encouraging kids to get up off the sofa and get active.

I love seeing the flow-on effect that Terri's focus on healthy living is having on her daughter. How else can we teach our children to be fit and healthy, unless we ourselves are living and breathing the very words that we preach? We cannot change a society that is facing escalating obesity concerns unless we educate the mothers who are responsible for raising the next generation. We need to show our kids how to entertain themselves at the park with a ball, on their bikes or in the swimming pool. We need to let them see us eating salads and vegetables with each meal and snacking on 'sports candy' such as carrots and fruit throughout the day.

This was the message with which Terri inspired the large gathering on the Sunshine Coast that day, and I was delighted to see a woman in her position using her power to reinforce messages of health and fitness to mums around the world. Terri does not aspire to be skinny, but rather to be a strong and healthy role model for her kids. That's powerful because her goals have nothing to do with the scales or a dress size, but are based around having the ability to do what needs to be done so she can live a life with no regrets.

I met Vickie's friends and caught up with her partner and two young boys who were there to see what Mum was doing. Vickie was very focused on her goal. She appeared on stage in the figure division, displaying an impressive amount of muscle and tone — she looked like someone who had been training for years, someone who I would assume had always been incredibly lean, fit and muscular. It was hard to believe that just a short while earlier I had met her when she was heavily pregnant and looking as curvy and voluptuous as you could imagine. She was unrecognisable standing up there on stage — I was absolutely blown away once again as I contemplated the amazing ability of our bodies to adapt and transform.

She stood proudly on stage, alongside the other female competitors — all kindred spirits in one way or another, in that they had concentrated a great deal of focus and energy on doing the work required to get to this point. I knew how much it would mean to Vickie if she was to walk away the winner, but I also felt as if just being up on that stage and belonging was an incredibly powerful place for her to be as well. I knew how devoted she was as a mum and I knew that she liked to challenge herself in ways that are outside her immediate role as a mother too. Here was the evidence that you can have it all in a sense — not that we all want to compete at this level, but it was an example of what is possible. Vickie might just as well have chosen to enter an art competition or stand on stage in a community theatre production — it really doesn't matter. What she had chosen to do was pursue a goal that was deeply meaningful to her, and she had succeeded in spectacular style.

Did Vickie walk away with the trophy that day? Unfortunately not. But to me she had already won the moment she set foot on stage. She had given it everything she had. She had proven to herself that she had what it took to be a serious contender, and whether or not it was enough for this particular judging panel was secondary to all that.

I walked away from the event with a newfound respect for people who explore the physical limits of our capabilities. Much as the experience of pregnancy had made me realise how pliable and limitless our physical bodies truly are, seeing these mothers (and grandmothers in some cases) on stage looking so toned and strong reinforced my belief that we are capable of so much more than we give ourselves credit for. We impose limits on ourselves where no limits actually exist. We stunt our growth and potential for joy by our own limited view of what is possible. We are limitless, constantly evolving, adaptive beings.

After this event I asked Kelli if she thought a mum who had never before been fit and healthy could really transform enough to compete at that level? To which Kelli replied, 'One hundred per cent yes! They can do it and I have seen it happen. Anything is possible, and it doesn't matter where you start from; it's only where you want to end up that counts.'

I have seen the women Kelli trains and I believe her when she says anything is possible. I cannot imagine her meeting someone and saying, 'Sorry love, but I just don't think your body is cut out for this looking and feeling good thing.' Kelli is just so incredibly positive about the potential that exists for all of us. It's hard to be around that kind of energy and not be changed by it.

Waking up with energy and being able to live my life to the max without relying on stimulants such as caffeine, sugar or fatty foods is incredibly rewarding. I love the feeling of control that comes with knowing what choices to make, and seeing the positive results flow out into every area of my life.

This is addiction at its best – fun, positive and life-enhancing!

Kelli shares her experience of working with Jodie

When Jodie first came to me it was all about seeing how her body could transform in the 12-week period. She was prepared to give it her all with diet and exercise. Like a lot of mums, Jodie was undereating, just picking at the leftovers from mealtimes or snacking on the crusts cut from sandwiches. She was leaving her main meal until dinner then going to bed on a full stomach and waking up with no energy. She did not drink anywhere near the recommended daily water intake, and this was another contributing factor to her lethargy.

Once Jodie started adding small things like protein shakes to her mid-morning and mid-afternoon snack time (instead of coffee and biscuits) her craving for sweet treats settled down and her metabolism started to speed up. Along with this I added starchy carbohydrates and protein for breakfast and lunch — carbohydrates in the form of oats, sweet potato, rice cakes and steamed rice, and protein in the form of eggs, fresh fish, tuna, steak, chicken and turkey — all good quality and lean!

To start with we kept the starchy carbohydrates out of the evening meal and replaced them with lots of fresh green vegetables or salad. Jodie began weight-training three times a week and did some form of cardio on most days — power walking, swimming or a run on the beach. Every week I took Jodie's measurements and changed her nutrition accordingly to keep the body fat coming off and check that she wasn't losing any lean muscle. Jodie is by no means a huge muscular woman but it is important to realise that you need lean muscle mass to assist in fat burning. As Jodie gained a little more muscle I increased the amounts of food and portion sizes to keep up with her metabolism. The bigger the engine, the more fuel it requires! As Jodie felt herself getting hungry every 2½ hours it was an indication that her metabolism was humming along nicely and that she was consuming the correct amount of calories to feed her muscles and burn the reserve stores of fat.

Jodie began to notice some very positive changes in her body. We could see more muscle definition, a tightened waistline and a more shapely body – not to mention increased energy and alertness.

Food is simply fuel for the body. Put the good quality fuel in and it will run at peak performance for you. It is important to be aware of what you are putting in your mouth and how it is affecting you. Jodie realised that her little snack of chocolate biscuits and caffeine every day would leave her feeling tired and craving another sugar pick-me-up shortly after the last. This is how the cycle starts, and it can easily get out of control.

Jodie is now taking much better care of herself and has the energy and vitality to ensure that she can give her all to her family and get the most out of life.

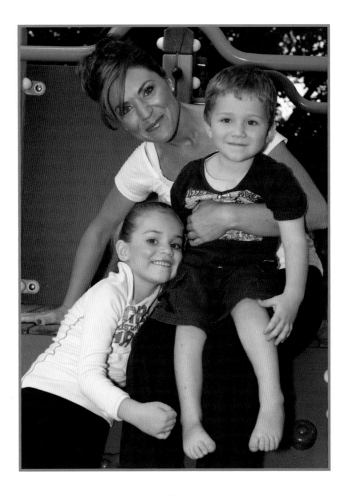

CASE STUDY

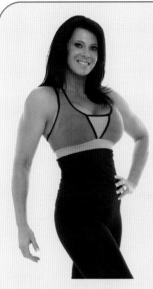

Kelli Johnson – mum, personal trainer and professional figure athlete

Kelli shares her journey towards fitness success at the highest levels internationally

Discover some interesting and rather surprising insights into Kelli's motherhood journey and how it acted as a catalyst for her embarking on a fitness career that now sees her competing around the world and training celebrity clients.

Kelli, tell us about your competition history and fitness achievements to date?

Most people are surprised to learn that I didn't actually start competing until after I had become a mum in my mid-thirties! It was my husband Colin, whom I met when my daughter Paige was quite young, who encouraged me to take my love of fitness to the next level and enter a figure competition. I won my very first competition as well as the first Miss Australia event I entered. I went on to compete in and then win the Miss Australasia title, and I knew pretty much straight away that this was something I was born to do! I am now very excited to have joined the IFBB Professional League, and am so excited to be competing on the international stage.

Did you study fitness?

Yes, I have a sport science degree and have been competing professionally and training others for over eight years now.

Were you always very active and health-conscious?

Yes, I have always been involved in sports – including gymnastics, equestrian, track and field.

Who were your early role models and what did they teach you?

I didn't have anyone who I can honestly say inspired me on my journey — fitness was more something I felt drawn towards, something that just made me feel good.

Who are your role models now — who teaches the teacher?

I am always inspired by the 'old-school' personal trainers — the basic principles have always worked and will continue to do so. I am always keeping up to date with the figure competitors in the US as this is where all major international and professional figure events are held. I also work with a couple of professional trainers overseas.

What is your motherhood story as it relates to fitness — how did motherhood affect you physically and emotionally?

During pregnancy I gained 22 kg! After the birth of my daughter I found it very difficult to settle into a routine. My daughter was a very unsettled baby, and I could not commit to my regular fitness regime. This was difficult for me as I began to feel there was less and less time available for me and I became totally consumed with looking after my child.

Emotionally I was suffering. I became depressed and developed irregular eating habits. I was sleep-deprived and couldn't find the time to keep myself physically fit. I was very unhappy with my body and my self-esteem suffered as a result.

Did you take time off being active after becoming a first-time mum?

Yes, I did take time off, as a result of looking after an unwell child. I remember my daughter would sleep for half an hour and then wake for an hour, around the clock constantly for three long months. I had no time or energy to be going to the gym or even getting outside to walk in the fresh air and sunlight — something I am now all too aware of as being one of the greatest energising sources we have available to us.

Was it difficult to regain focus and control of your body?

Initially it was difficult as I had been skipping meals and regular mealtimes were a thing of the past. This was the biggest challenge – to eat small meals more often instead of picking at food I was preparing for my daughter, like the crust cut from a sandwich or leftovers from her meal. Believe it or not, this does become a habit and it does creep up on you.

How much of an impact do you think exercise had on your experience in overcoming post-natal depression (PND)?

For me personally, exercise was the single most beneficial tool of all the therapies that I tried to overcome PND. The fact that I got up, went outside and walked in the sunlight and fresh air gave me a new lease of life. Then as I began feeling more confident and energised I made my way to a gym and began training with weights again. This change of events started the wonderful process of producing the feel-good hormones, endorphins – which were something I had lacked for quite some time! Before I knew it I was starting to feel strong again and my fitness levels were returning. I was beginning to get more and better quality sleep and my appetite was returning.

Did you go on antidepressants and, if so, did you feel comfortable with this decision?

Yes, my doctor recommended that I try antidepressants; however, I soon discovered that they were not the right choice for me. That experience led me to try things that would assist my body and mind in returning to health naturally. I made the choice to nourish my body through dietary changes and a regular fitness program along with a revised time-management program that allowed me to rest, eat and work out on a regular basis. Consistency was, and still is, the key.

What does a typical week look like for you in terms of training?

It's different depending on whether I am working towards a competition or not. Typically my week consists of four weight-training sessions and five dedicated cardio sessions. At weekends I am always involved with family and that usually takes us to the beach where we do active stuff like surfing or swimming. When I am preparing for a competition, I step up to five weight-training sessions and seven dedicated cardio days.

How do you keep up your training and good nutrition when travelling?

When I travel I always stick to the basic nutritional principles I promote. I try to eat as fresh and 'clean' as possible – which means avoiding highly processed convenience food. As far as training goes I generally find a gym or I will make use of an outdoor area such as a park or running track/football field and use my own body-weight to create resistance.

Do you worry about your weight and the scales?

No, I never use the scales as an indicator of how I am doing with my weight. Muscle weighs more than fat and the scales don't tell you what your muscle/fat ratio is. I think scales can mess with your head, especially when you are training hard and on a great nutritional program – you would expect to see them go down, but usually they don't as we gain a little more muscle mass when we are training and eating correctly.

What keeps you motivated to continue working out?

I am motivated to exercise daily as it makes me feel good. I like knowing that my immune system is strong and that I can keep up with the kids! It's great to feel comfortable in my clothes, but I am not the smallest size and never will be. I am happy in my skin and like to be the best I can without comparing myself to magazine covers or trying to follow any trends for body image.

What has been the hardest challenge on your health and fitness journey?

I would have to say the hardest thing as a professional figure athlete would be taking the dieting to the next level. It is very strict and I am usually competing in the first three months of the year, which means I am on my training diet throughout Christmas and New Year. This is when all the best food is around, but I just tell myself that I have made the choice and no one is forcing me to do this, so just get on with it! My weakness would have to be banana smoothies and donuts. Yum!

Was there ever a time when you weren't the super-fit athlete we see today?

Yes, I wasn't always as fit as I am now. I had to be very realistic about what I could achieve after my daughter was born and I certainly didn't have the same amount of time to dedicate to the gym. I was happy when I started making a concerted effort to go outside every day and walk and breathe in the fresh air. Happy just to be swimming and burning off the extra calories I had consumed by picking at foods that weren't good for me. Fitness is something that is gained by being consistent and dedicated. A little every day will get you on your way!

What do you do to continually inspire and motivate yourself — any tips for us mums?

I like to read good health and fitness magazines — my personal favourites are *Oxygen* and *Muscle and Fitness* — they always have great tips on training and nutrition. I am also inspired by my wonderful clients, all of whom bring amazing stories to my life — watching them transform their lives in so many ways while working together gives me the ultimate joy.

What is your favourite book?

My favourite book would have to be *The Secret*, along with the movie of the same title. I am a great believer in the saying 'thoughts become things'!

Any key moments in your life that affected you in a big way and made you the woman you are today?

Yes, the moment I realised that in order to be a good mother and keep up with my daughter for the many years ahead, I would have to become physically, emotionally and mentally fit … and the only person who could make this happen was ME!

**Mums always complain they are too tired/busy to exercise —
what do you say to them?**

Sick and tired of being sick and tired … nothing is going to change with that attitude! Make some simple changes and stick to them. Don't be too proud to ask for help if you need someone to look after your baby or children while you go to the gym or out for a walk — you will be amazed at what some time out will do for your head-space and fitness. Start eating regularly and if you need to sleep during the day then do it when your child rests — the chores will wait. If you aren't getting enough sleep, everything else will start to fall apart. You will find you are able to give more quality time to your family when you have taken some time for yourself.

Where would you like to see yourself in ten years, Kelli — what's in the future for you?

Happy, fit and healthy and still helping others reach their personal goals in life.

Proudest health and fitness moment?

My career highlights would be winning Miss Australia twice, representing Australia at the world titles and becoming a professional athlete in my forties.

What advice would you give to mums who want to pursue a healthier lifestyle — what are the first steps you would recommend?

Find a trainer or fitness professional who walks the talk and can give you experienced advice on training and proper nutrition. Get a plan that will realistically fit into your schedule and do something outside every day.

Final words of inspiration?

I like this one —

*Why wait? Life is not a dress rehearsal. Quit practising what you
are going to do, and just do it!*
UNKNOWN

Introducing the

International Motherhood Study

(Australia & New Zealand)

The International Motherhood Study (IMS) launched on Mother's Day 2009 and became one of the largest studies focusing on the emotional journey of a mother ever undertaken.

Directly inspired by the response to my book, *You Sexy Mother — a life-changing approach to motherhood*, the study's primary aim was to explore the emotional landscape of motherhood — essentially to get inside the mind, body and soul of as many mums as possible in order to truly understand how it feels to be a mum today.

By the end of 2009, a total of 4708 women across Australia and New Zealand had each completed 131 questions relating to their motherhood journey via the anonymous on-line survey at www.motherhoodstudy.net

Relevant health and fitness-related findings from the study have been inserted alongside key messages within this book, with the aim of providing a reference point to help you better appreciate your own relationship with your body.

The statistics shown in boxes throughout this book have been calculated on the basis of the responses of 4708 women across Australia and New Zealand. At the time of writing, a full analysis of data is being carried out by statisticians and full disclosure of the key findings will follow from there.

Statistics serve a purpose, but they have limited obvious benefits to most of us in our day-to-day life. It is my hope, however, that showing you the emerging trends and allowing you to work out where you sit alongside the mums surveyed will transform the way you look at the importance of health and fitness in your life.

The number of mums who were surveyed is overwhelming and the results are compelling. Look out for the research boxes (with blue type) throughout the book for more information.

Thank you to each and every woman who contributed her story.

With every rising of the sun,
Think of your life as just begun
UNKNOWN

THE INTERNATIONAL MOTHERHOOD STUDY

Exercise patterns (before, during and after pregnancy)

We can see from the results of the study that pregnancy and the transition into motherhood have a significant impact on exercise trends for women. Prior to pregnancy, a large number of the women (57%) reported that they exercised a minimum of three to four times per week. During pregnancy only 39% of them continued to exercise at this level, and following pregnancy the percentage increases a modest 3% to just 42%.

This shows that almost 60% of mothers are not taking sufficient exercise to receive the associated health benefits of regular exercise.

	Before pregnancy	During pregnancy	After pregnancy
Exercise daily	18%	11%	12%
3-4 x per week	38% = 56%	28% = 39%	30% = 42%
Once a week	16%	25%	22%
Do not exercise regularly	28%	36%	36%

Of the women who did exercise regularly prior to pregnancy (at least three or four times a week), approximately 60% continued with regular exercise during pregnancy and after childbirth. Almost 70% of the mothers who exercised daily continued with a regime of at least regular exercise after birth. This compares to just 30% of the women who did not exercise regularly before pregnancy.

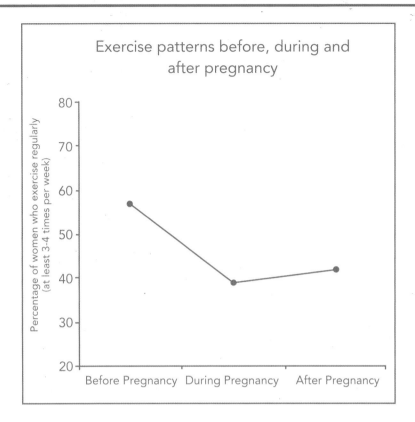

Exercise patterns before, during and after pregnancy

In short, if you exercise regularly before pregnancy, you are about twice as likely to exercise regularly after pregnancy. We can also see that one in three of the women who did not exercise regularly before pregnancy did go on to be regular exercisers as mothers.

What is interesting to note is that while we might expect the number of mums who exercise regularly to decline during pregnancy, there is very little change in our exercise patterns as we move from pregnancy into early motherhood and beyond. We appear to adopt a certain level of exercise, or non-exercise, behaviour during pregnancy, and then maintain that as our life moves forward.

As the full analysis of the data unfolds, we will be able to look at these exercise patterns for mums in terms of their age, number of children and associated factors such as levels of support they receive and experience of post-natal depression.

For now, these numbers indicate that many women are adopting a set point regarding exercise, which appears to have been created during pregnancy.

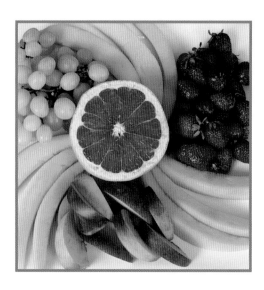

Body Bible Basics:

Nutrition

Ten Success Principles

Simple fact: You are in control of what you eat. That's it. Put this statement everywhere —
look at it before every morsel you eat. Especially when you are eating alone and between meals.
Those are the times we hide — trying hardest to hide from ourselves as well as others.

DR ANGELA HUNTSMAN

The following principles are exactly what I learnt during my 12 weeks working with Kelli. They are what she teaches every woman who enters her home training studio and the fabulously fit and healthy world in which she lives!

It was a long journey to get there, but once I discovered and then applied this magic formula, weight that had clung to me like a new-born baby evaporated before my very eyes.

The good news is — I know it will work for you too!

1. Nutrition *is* the secret

Nutrition + training = Fast track to success
Training alone is not enough.

So often we see or hear about people who go to the gym almost every day but show no tangible results for their efforts. I know I have been there myself in the past – working alongside a trainer and achieving mediocre gains at best. I don't know about you, but if I am going to hit the gym on a regular basis I want to start seeing some mind-blowing results! What I have learnt from researching this topic and talking to fitness experts is that very often personal trainers focus only on the training, never even discussing how nutrition fits into the big picture.

That's like telling someone that the pot of gold really does exist at the end of the rainbow, without telling them where the rainbow is and how they can reach the end of it. To really see the kind of results I know you are looking for, you need to understand how your body processes food and what the consequences will be for each of the food choices you make.

That way you can choose when and how you eat and be in a position of personal power. You'll know important information like the fact that a meal high in carbohydrates consumed late at night has nowhere else to go (in a biochemical sense) than attach itself to our accumulated fat stores on our thighs, stomach, back (yikes!) or upper arms, to name but a few obvious destinations. It's not the carbs' fault – they are just doing what they have to do because there is no physical exertion taking place at that time of day to use up the energy they have just provided.

A bowl of oats eaten first thing in the morning, however (my breakfast of choice, with honey and sultanas) will be well utilised by your body after a morning power walk around the neighbourhood. The same bowl of oats eaten at a different time of day will produce a completely different outcome. The wonderful thing about nutrition is that once you understand how powerful it is in terms of being able to support or sabotage your health and fitness efforts, you can use it to generate unbelievable changes in your body in less time than you would believe. The power lies in knowledge, and arming yourself with enough of it to help you achieve your goals (without overloading yourself to the point of total confusion). So we will give it to you simply and concisely – everything you need to know and nothing you don't.

2. Eat more, not less

Eat six times throughout the day, every three hours, from the time you wake up.
How excited are you as you read that?

Eat more not less – is this healthy living making Jodie a little nutty? I admit my new diet does incorporate a good dose of nuts now and then, but fortunately it has improved my mental capabilities, not the other way round, and yes, you did read right – this 'diet' is about eating more of the good stuff and resisting the urge to skip meals in the false belief that it will help you look the way you want.

I admit that I was one of those mums who was guilty of skipping meals in the hope that it would help me stay slim. I would often gobble down a couple of cookies with my coffee and call that a meal for the next three to four hours. It wasn't making me fat, but it was turning me into a 'skinny fat' mum at best (relatively slender, but saggy and baggy). I was relying on sugar and caffeine to give me a false sense of the energy I so desperately wanted to enjoy. The reality is that after a few weeks on the new eating plan I was enjoying more food and certainly more meals each day, yet the excess weight (or in my case fat) felt like it was slipping off my body, revealing a sexier, healthier and, most important, more energetic me!

3. Your body loves routine

Your body needs to believe that there is no shortage of food.
If we reflect on the seasons and the concept of time, the tides, the moon and almost every aspect of our lives, we can see how our universe is governed by a degree of regularity and routine that is nothing short of miraculous. Is it any wonder then that part of the secret to taking control of your physical body rests with the concept of establishing a good routine?

Why then do so many of us women still adhere to the skipping-breakfast mentality and cling to the false premise that a skipped meal here and there will mean that an overindulgence some other time will go unnoticed by our bodies? You would think we should know better by now, but to be honest, this was still a concept that I had to really work hard to embrace as I too was guilty of thinking that skipping the odd meal had allowed me to eat pretty much what I wanted the rest of the time.

Kelli put me straight the very first day we met – 'Our bodies love routine, Jodie!' she announced. When you skip meals your body is always in feast-or-famine mode and will continue to store energy (yes, as fat!) for those times when you skip meals and it thinks there are no longer any calories available. To switch your body into a fat-burning machine you need to constantly reassure it (by eating every three hours) that there is no threat of famine and therefore no reason to store excess energy. This regular eating pattern creates a body that learns to operate like an efficient machine – absorbing energy, utilising that energy to do all the bodily functions required and then burning off any additional energy during the day. There is no need for large reserves to be gathered as it has been 'trained' (by you) to know that food is plentiful and will be arriving frequently to fulfil all necessary requirements.

4. Don't be scared of the carbs

Carbs are not the enemy, we just need to know how to make them work for us. There is so much fear and negativity surrounding carbohydrates these days that you could be forgiven for thinking they are the body's worst enemy. The public success of programs such as the Atkins Diet (which severely restricted carb intake) has led many people to avoid carbohydrates when in fact they are still an important ally if you want to look and feel great. They provide us with valuable energy that is steadily released throughout the day as well as many mood-enhancing properties that are important on so many levels as a mum. To exclude them completely is not only unnecessary but also counter-productive to creating the high-energy results we are promoting here.

The golden rule with carbs is to consume them early or consume them prior to exercise. If you load up early in the day, you have a long time in which to be active and use up the energy they provide. If, on the other hand, you effectively starve yourself all day then tuck into a huge calorie-laden bowl of your favourite creamy pasta at night, your body has *no choice* but to store the carbs as fat, for a time when your body does need extra energy – like when the next potato famine hits town! Unfortunately for your waistline, you will more than likely consume enough calories the next day to meet your current energy requirements, so that pasta meal that stuck so quickly and joyfully to your hips is there to stay, my friend.

Knowledge is power, as they say, and that is why some people seem to be able to eat everything and never gain a pound while others struggle their whole lives to make sense of it all. Here's another top tip … we need to be careful about the type of carbohydrate we consume.

Starchy carbs are the low GI ones you read about — GI stands for glycemic index, and basically refers to whether something is a 'slow-burn' or a 'fast-burn' food. If it is low GI, it will give you a slow, steady release of energy and keep you feeling full for longer — good news for those of us pursuing a healthy body and lifestyle. So fuel up on choices such as sweet potato, brown rice, rye bread and rolled oats for a healthy dose of carbs, and look at reducing (then eliminating!) anything made with refined sugar, white rice, white bread … all very high GI, fast-releasing energy foods. You will get an immediate burst of energy, followed by a big low, where your body naturally begins to look for the next 'hit' in the form of a sugary carbohydrate snack such as a muffin or chocolate biscuit. This is a vicious cycle (trust me, I know first-hand) and one you want to exit from as quickly as possible.

5. Water — your secret weapon

**You need 8+ glasses of water per day minimum —
more if you are exercising and during the summer.**

Water is absolutely critical to the success of any weight-management program. It can make the difference between reaching your goals and ending up sabotaging your success along the way.

I cannot overemphasise the importance of this miracle substance! It's up to you whether you want to buy bottled water, use a purifier or drink it straight from the tap — there is so much contradictory advice about which is best, and that is not the focus of this book. All I know from studying alongside Kelli and my research is that water is the equivalent of a wonder drug, so get it into you any way you can!

Water will be your best ally as you embark on your body transformation — helping you feel fuller for longer, keeping you feeling sharp and energetic, reducing the incidence of headaches and helping you fight off colds and flu. Additional benefits include flushing out toxins and keeping your skin radiant — what more could you ask for?

Don't be fooled into thinking that eight cups of tea and coffee will do the trick — it won't, as they actually have a slight diuretic effect and can make you more dehydrated.

Remember the simple rule — if it looks pretty much the same on the way out as it did going in (think clear, not yellow!), you are doing well. If not, increase your water intake accordingly.

Not rocket science, just common sense … You can do this!

WATER AND WEIGHT LOSS

Research has proven conclusively that insufficient water intake results in excess body fat, poor muscle tone, digestive complications, muscle soreness and, ironically, water-retention problems.

When you consider that a normal adult's body is 60-70% water, it's easy to see why this is the most important element for survival. We can go without food for almost two months, but without water only a few days. Many of us have no idea how much water we need to drink and as a result live in a constantly dehydrated state.

By consuming the recommended eight to ten glasses of water throughout the day, you could be on your way to a healthier, leaner body. If people who are trying to lose weight don't drink enough water, their body can't metabolise the fat adequately. Retaining fluid will also keep your weight high.

You should spread your intake throughout the day and evening. Many people worry that if they drink the recommended amount they will be running to the bathroom all day. In reality, this might be the case for the first few weeks, but after a while your bladder tends to adjust.

Health benefits of drinking water include:
- Regulates appetite
- Metabolism increases
- Energy levels are boosted
- Less water retention and 'bloating'
- Alleviates headaches
- Reduces blood pressure
- Reduces high cholesterol
- Eases joint pain
- Decreases risk of certain cancers
- Reduces chance of developing kidney stones
- Releases toxic waste products
- Improves skin

6. Protein is king

A diet rich in protein is essential. Feeding your muscles will assist in weight loss. This is how it works – and trust me, this one principle has totally revolutionised the way I eat (and look).

Muscles need to be fed or they will disappear. If you think about it like that, it makes it simple. You may not want to look like a body builder (and you won't, unless you work very hard at it), but it's good to look after your muscles because the more muscle you have, relative to fat, the more your body will burn calories even while you sleep. That's great news for anyone who wants to be able to enjoy food *and* look fabulous.

Including adequate protein in your diet (with most meals) will help your body to switch over to burning excess fat stores for energy instead of burning muscle for energy. This is true for anyone who combines regular protein intake with a dedicated fitness program and a balanced nutritional plan.

If you are increasing your daily protein intake you will need to increase your daily water intake also. Metabolising protein requires more water than fats or carbohydrates, so adjust your intake accordingly.

Good protein sources include fresh fish, chicken, turkey, red meat, eggs and nuts. The portion size for fish, chicken and meat should be around 100-120 g (this is roughly the size of the palm of your hand). You can have slightly more with fish. Protein tends to take longer to process and will give you a feeling of satiety for longer after each meal.

So while you might find it difficult at first to replace your biscuits with rice cakes topped with peanut butter, or cottage cheese and chicken breast, you will feel much fuller for longer and will find that you no longer need the sugary fix like before.

Good sources of protein for vegetarians include chickpeas, beans, tofu, lentils, eggs, nuts and seeds.

7. Sugar *not* fat is the enemy

Sugar can wreak havoc with your ability to maintain a healthy weight, and with your emotional well-being. Refined sugar is bad for you because it raises the insulin level in your blood. Raised blood insulin levels depress the immune system. If your immune system is depressed then your ability to fight disease is weakened.

Sugar gives you a quick pick-me-up but will also leave you feeling flat and tired shortly after. Calories from sugar that are not used during exercise or daily activity will be stored in the body as fat. If you look carefully and read your food labels you will see that most diet and 'light' products contain more sugar than the regular option. In order to make them a 'diet' product, the fat is taken out and often replaced with more sugar. These products appear to be healthier but you need to be aware of what the sugar is doing to your system. The following are just some of the repercussions for your system from consuming excess sugar:

· Suppresses the immune system
· Upsets the body's mineral balance
· Speeds the ageing process, causing wrinkles and grey hair
· Increases total cholesterol
· Contributes to weight gain and obesity
· Contributes to diabetes
· Causes food allergies
· Can cause toxemia during pregnancy
· May cause depression
· Increases the body's fluid retention
· May cause hormonal imbalance
· May cause headaches, including migraines

Lifestyle recommendations

It is very important that you look to reduce stress in as many areas of your life as possible. Exercise is extremely beneficial, as is eating regularly and often – including nutrient-rich foods at every opportunity.

Nutrient-rich foods for blood sugar balance:

· **Vitamin C**
  Citrus fruits, kiwifruit, sprouted seeds, blackcurrants, tomatoes and peppers.
· **B-complex**
  Eggs, game, pumpkin seeds, blackstrap molasses, wheatgerm, brewers' yeast.
· **Chromium**
  Egg yolk, molasses, brewers' yeast, fruit, whole grains and nuts.
· **Magnesium**
  Fish, lentils, nuts and seeds, dried fruits and green leafy vegetables.
· **Zinc**
  The richest food sources are oysters, liver, brewers' yeast, eggs, whole grains, pumpkin seeds and mushrooms.

BLOOD SUGAR IMBALANCE

Blood sugar imbalance is a serious condition relating to your body's inability to handle glucose effectively. Throughout the day blood glucose levels can fluctuate outside the body's desired range. They may go from being very high after a meal, stimulant or stress, to being very low, if for example you skipped breakfast. Insulin is the hormone responsible for keeping the blood sugar levels within the normal desired range. It works by opening channels on cell membranes, allowing glucose to travel from the blood into the cells.

Blood sugar imbalance can be a precursor to diabetes and it is vital that people who consider themselves to be at risk establish a healthy lifestyle and address any contributory factors before the condition develops further.

Warning signs you may experience due to a blood sugar imbalance include:
· Needing more than eight hours' sleep
· Feeling thirsty
· Needing coffee or tea to get you going
· Frequent urination
· Heavy sweating regularly during the day
· Fatigue
· Dizziness
· Mood swings
· Cravings for sweet foods
· Headaches
· Palpitations
· Energy dips

Fats are often thought about only in negative terms, but they provide energy, maintain body temperature, insulate nerves, and cushion and protect body tissues. Most foods contain several different kinds of fats — including saturated, polyunsaturated, monounsaturated and trans fats — and some kinds are better for your health than others.

You don't need to completely eliminate all fats from your meals. Instead, choose the healthier types of fats and enjoy them in moderation.

Type of healthy fat:	Food source:
Monounsaturated fat	Olive oil, peanut oil, canola oil, avocados, nuts and seeds
Polyunsaturated fat	Vegetable oils (such as safflower, corn, sunflower, soy and cottonseed oils), nuts and seeds
Omega-3 fatty acids	Fatty, cold-water fish (such as salmon, mackerel and herring), flaxseeds, flax oil and walnuts

ESSENTIAL FATTY ACID DEFICIENCY

Good fats such as flaxseed oil are known as essential fatty acids, and the body needs them to make hormones and maintain its metabolic rate. A deficiency in these good oils can cause cravings, especially for fatty foods.

If you think you may be deficient, watch out for signs such as dandruff, dry hair and dry, scaly skin. Deficiency is also associated with arthritis, eczema, heart disease, diabetes and premenstrual syndrome.

8. Supplements

When you start eating 'clean', reducing refined foods and consuming more fruit, vegetables and lean protein, you reduce the need for excessive supplementation.

Although we try to eat a variety of fresh and healthy foods, our nutritional requirements are often still not met by our food choices. The following supplements are what Kelli recommends her clients consider to help bring their energy levels and immunity up to peak performance levels:

- **A good multivitamin**
  A good daily multivitamin/mineral supplement improves your overall bodily functioning and boosts both your physical and mental health and well-being.

- **Omega-3**

Omega-3 fatty acids are essential, meaning they are necessary to your health, but the body is unable to produce them. They must be obtained from the diet. Research shows that supplementation of Omega-3 can help prevent heart disease, maintain optimum blood pressure and cholesterol levels, and give almost immediate relief from joint pain, migraines, depression, autoimmune diseases and many other conditions.

Omega-3 has also been shown to improve people's ability to concentrate and to think more clearly in general – the perfect brain food. Omega-3/fish oil is also highly recommended by nearly every well-respected diet/fitness/nutrition expert of any kind as one of the few supplements that should be taken by anyone with the goal of building muscle, losing fat, or improving their fitness level or athletic ability.

- **Magnesium**

Magnesium is needed for more than 300 biochemical reactions in the body. It helps maintain normal muscle and nerve function, and keeps heart rhythm steady and bones strong. It is also involved in energy metabolism and protein synthesis.

- **Calcium**

As well as assisting in the prevention of osteoporosis, calcium is required for blood coagulation, nerve function, production of energy, the beating of the heart, proper immune function and muscle contraction.

- **Protein powder and protein bars (optional)**

Incorporating protein powder and protein bars into your diet is completely optional and is not required in order to see dramatic changes over time. However, for many of us mums (myself included), they can be a great morning- and afternoon-tea option and save you skipping meals during those times when you are at work or out and about with the kids.

I take my pre-measured powder in a small container along with a shaker filled with a cup of water. I can just add my chocolate protein powder to my shaker and instantly enjoy a chocolaty treat – knowing that it is fuelling my body and helping me to avoid reaching for high-sugar, high-fat snacks instead. A protein bar in your bag can help you avoid reaching for a muffin or cookie every time you feel hungry and need something to tide you over until you get home. Protein powders are made from four basic sources: whey (from milk), egg, soy and rice. They can also be a combination of one or more ingredients. These concentrated sources of protein are processed into the powdered form, to be reconstituted into liquid form as a protein shake when mixed with water, fruit juice or milk. Most protein powders are fortified with other nutrients such as amino acids, vitamins and minerals, all of which are essential for health. Ask your health store professional for guidance when deciding which option is best for you.

9. Don't beat up on yourself

Make it a habit to disconnect good and bad with food. It's just … food.
ANDERS LINDGREEN

There is just no way you can stop and start a healthy lifestyle program based on doing 'good or bad' each day and hope to achieve long-term success. Your attitude needs to reflect the idea that each day we start anew, and each day we need to recommit to living a healthy, high-energy lifestyle. The odd indulgence is all part of a healthy balanced approach to life, and certainly not something to beat yourself up over.

Social events and celebrations are a wonderful part of life, and Kelli's advice to me was to just make the best choices I could nutritionally in each moment. She reminded me that it wouldn't be perfect, no matter what I chose, but that I still needed to be able to live a full and fun life and this was part of my learning. I realised that there were times when I could say no to dessert, but there were also occasions like family celebrations when saying no to a slice of cake just didn't feel right and would be taking things too far. So I said yes and no as each occasion presented itself, and soon worked out that it wasn't the cake or dessert that was the problem – it was my reaction the next day that had the power to really make or break my commitment to my new lifestyle program.

I had to learn to wake up and get my running shoes on regardless of whether or not I ate cake the night before. That was a difficult lesson to learn as we can get so used to punishing ourselves for not being 'perfect' and sabotaging our success by giving up just when the results are about to shine through. Kelli's top quote to keep in mind in this situation is:

Give up the guilt. People make mistakes, and so will you. It's okay to move on. Never let yesterday use up today. Your future is ahead of you, not behind you.

UNKNOWN

10. The 80:20 rule applies

Most of us have heard of the 80:20 rule and how it has been proven to be effective in so many areas of our lives — like the fact that 80% of our joy in life comes from 20% of the activities we engage in. We can incorporate this simple concept into our search for a better body in a very powerful and empowering way. All we need to do is stick to the nutrition and exercise principles outlined in this book 80% of the time, so we can afford to be less than perfect for the other 20% of the time with little or indeed no negative outcome.

How liberating! So the next time you overindulge at a Christmas party or enjoy some hot chips by the seaside with the family, just chalk it up as your 20% and resolve not to let it hold you back in your quest to experience optimal health and fitness. I recall reading about certain supermodels who would eat and exercise diligently six days of the week and then indulge in whatever they wanted every Sunday — it's just another example of the 80:20 rule at work — even Kelli agrees it is okay (and indeed healthy) to look at your week like this. It will probably mean you are less likely to go way off-track as a result of one little deviation, and your chances of achieving long-term results that last will be far greater.

As a wise woman once said to me many years ago:

Jodie, if you are going to do something and feel guilty about it, then don't do it. But if you do decide to do it, don't waste a minute of your life feeling guilty about it!

This was a woman who was so incredibly comfortable in her own skin – on every level. She had integrity, values and a deep sense of being guided by her own light. What a wonderful lesson she taught me, and it's one that resonates every day as I continue on my quest for optimal health and well-being.

Finally, a note about alcohol …

Alcohol is almost as energy-dense as fat and is often accompanied by sugary drinks. The liver processes the alcohol, and whenever there is any of it in your system it gets priority over converting fat into energy. Every mouthful is effectively halting your fat-burning activities for hours.

The bottom line is that you have to know the effect that alcohol is having on your body. A little of a good thing is a truly good thing. But just don't overdo it, because it will not only give your body an immediate high-calorie hit (and stop your fat-burning activities for a good while) but there's no question it will be affecting your ability to make good food choices in the hours or day following any binge.

Look to reduce if not eliminate alcohol for the first few weeks of your body transformation program, just to give yourself the best possible chance of success. After that you can incorporate a moderate amount into a healthy lifestyle, simply by being honest about what it is doing to your body and thinking of it much as you would any treat or celebration food.

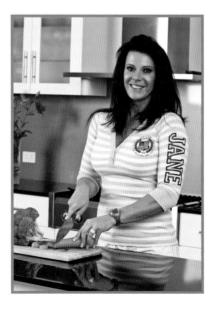

FOOD ALLERGIES

Have you ever eaten something — a bowl of ice cream, chocolate, a slice of bread — and felt even hungrier than before? Are there certain foods that you crave, and you find it difficult to satisfy that craving?

A 'yes' to the questions above could indicate a food allergy. If you also struggle to lose weight, then it is possible that this allergy is contributing to your weight issue.

Food sensitivities are difficult to combat as they cause people to crave the very foods to which they are allergic. Just as a caffeine addict experiences withdrawal symptoms when they stop drinking coffee (usually in the form of headaches), allergic people experience discomfort when they can no longer eat a particular food.

Sugar addiction leads people to consume large amounts of sugar to make themselves feel good. Much like drug addicts, there are sugar addicts, and I think many mums can relate to this addiction to varying degrees. In my research for this book I read an alarming case study of a woman who would eat a tablespoon of sugar as soon as her husband left for work, because it would make her feel good — she would actually get high on sugar. Three or four hours later this same woman would go into a depression, and she had attempted suicide several times. These suicide attempts were prompted by withdrawal symptoms. This woman didn't get well until her doctor established a food allergy connection. Now she realises that she must read the ingredient lists on all food labels.

I have seen first-hand the change in my son after he stopped eating wheat and gluten following his diagnosis of coeliac disease. He went from being a very poorly fussy eater, with a distended stomach and inexplicable weight loss, to a thriving little boy who now loves to eat his vegetables and looks a picture of good health. Not only did he improve physically, but his emotional well-being became more stable — with none of the highs and lows in mood that existed prior to his diagnosis.

Food allergies are serious and can have major implications for our ability to live a full and vital life. If you feel you may be sensitive to certain foods and want more information, visit your doctor and ask to be referred to a specialist.

Kelli's kitchen tips & tricks

First up, here's the good news — **Kelli loves her food!**

Yes, even a top fitness trainer and professional figure athlete like my friend Kelli enjoys her food. What is even more interesting (and incredibly comforting) is that she admits her weakness is donuts. Donuts, donuts, donuts … she swears she could eat 12 in a sitting! But rest assured, Kelli has tips and tricks that allow her to resist doing that (too often!) and instead maintain her awesome body and optimal state of health.

Would you like to know how to avoid the sugar-trap every day? You know, the one that hits most of us mums around mid-afternoon … normally it's when you are busy trying to do the school pick-up, or during that fussy baby period that rattles you to the core before dinnertime. I know I did, as sugar and I (or should I say chocolate and I, to be more specific) had been friends for a long time up until I met Kelli, and I really wanted to know how I could give up this addiction without feeling total desperation.

Kelli conducts a wonderful and enlightening course for clients in her home, where she shares all her hard-earned kitchen secrets about how to prepare flavoursome food that is good for you, along with how to get organised so eating well is a breeze. Today I signed up for her course and this is what I learnt …

This girl is organised

While it didn't surprise me to see how organised Kelli is when it comes to preparing her food in advance, what did amaze me was how quick and simple it was to prepare food for my whole family for the next two or three days. Kelli gave me a simple shopping list before my class that included basic items I could source from the supermarket. And believe it or not, there wasn't a can of tuna in sight.

Kelli told me that one of her aims in life is to show people that eating well does not mean you have to exist on tins of tuna and salad day after day. She chatted away as she took 500 g of sliced chicken breast and marinated it briefly with chopped fresh garlic, a whole squeezed lemon, chopped basil and coriander, along with some salt and pepper and a drizzle of good oil (macadamia or coconut oil is great). The smell was exquisite, with the basil energising us as we cooked, and before I knew it we had some delicious, flavoursome chicken pieces that could be put into a rice bread wrap with salad for lunch along with a drizzle of natural yogurt, or served with vegetables or salad for a tasty dinner.

I was actually surprised Kelli added any oil, as you hear so much about fat being the enemy of anyone looking to have a great body. 'Oil is a good fat,' Kelli said. 'It's refined sugar and starchy carbs that really mess with your body, not the good oils like avocado and nuts.' She explained that she is very wary of buying 'low-fat' products, since the manufacturers often add a lot of sugar and the carbohydrate content is higher. Kelli's philosophy is that it is better to have a little of the real thing than to pour low-fat alternatives into your body en masse. Think a drizzle of honey on your cereal instead of spoonfuls of sugar, or some natural Greek yogurt with your chicken and salad wrap — that's how she does it. It also means you get to have some 'goodies' in a moderate, balanced way, rather than feeling completely deprived of the good stuff day after day.

To make your vegetables more flavoursome, try seasoning them liberally with fresh herbs such as basil and coriander during the steaming process (steaming is infinitely better than boiling all of the goodness out of them).

The other delicious treat we whipped up for my family was lean mince patties, made both healthy and flavoursome in minutes. We combined 500 g of mince with tomato paste and flavouring (you can use any chilli or satay-style seasoning you like depending on how hot you want it). We mixed it to a good consistency then formed patties which we fried in a non-stick pan. These patties are tasty for the whole family and can be used in a wrap, with salad, or you can take the cooked mincemeat and add cucumber, red pepper and fresh herbs then wrap it all in a lettuce leaf, for something a little different.

For a chicken mince alternative, try combining 500 g of chicken with half a tub of Greek yogurt, toasted pinenuts, chopped fresh coriander and some salt and pepper. These make delicious patties too, or the mixture can be cooked up as chicken mince and added to a wrap with some peanut butter for extra protein and flavour — delicious.

The options are limitless, and I walked away from Kelli's house with enough food to keep me and my family satisfied for the next couple of days at least.

Key discoveries from Kelli's 'Kitchen Tips & Tricks' session

Think twice, act once

A powerful reminder Kelli gives to her clients is the idea that they should always stop and think about their food choices before shopping or putting anything into their bodies. That way, the journey will be much quicker and more rewarding, simply because you have presence of mind when shopping for or preparing food. Never go to the supermarket on an empty stomach — the temptation to buy too much of the wrong foods will be too great. It is worth mentioning, too, that shopping with little ones can be extremely distracting and challenging at times, so to begin with organise some assistance so you can get to the shops on your own a couple of times — that way you'll be able to read the food labels and check out healthy options. Once you have a new plan and list ready to go, then you can bring along the kids — just give yourself a fighting start in those first few weeks. I did a couple of night excursions after putting my little ones to bed and found it was really helpful. It was so quiet and calm that I was able to read labels and find things that I don't normally even see as I am dashing about.

Milk products

Like many mums, I like a bit of dairy. Milk in my tea, the occasional yogurt, an icecream on a hot day at the beach. Kelli explained that dairy is not well tolerated by many of us and is known to be a leading cause of food allergies in both children and adults. So how does she resist the dairy trap in a bid to look and feel great? 'Dash' is the word she uses. Put a dash of milk in, not half a cup, when making your tea, coffee or hot chocolate. In fact, I found a delicious hot chocolate drink mix in her cupboards, which she makes up with water. Instead of the recommended 3 tbsp of powder, Kelli worked out that she could use half that amount and still create a delicious hot chocolate drink to enjoy whenever she feels the need for a little something sweet. It's all about moderation.

Prepare in advance

Kelli recommends preparing food two or three times during the week, so you never get to the point where there is nothing in the fridge and you resort to buying takeaways and expensive meals that you don't have control over. You can never really be sure what is going into your takeaway food or how fresh the ingredients are. As your system grows accustomed to predominantly fresh, healthy food, your body is less able to tolerate fast food, and it is likely to give you a sore stomach and a bloated feeling. The added bonus of always having food to hand is that you save money on takeaways, and no longer find yourself wasting money on snacks when out and about.

We always have choices

Keep in mind the fact that we always have choices. Ask yourself, What alternatives do I have right now? I could have a chocolate bar or I could make a delicious energy shake with honey, natural peanut butter, LSA (ground linseed, sunflower seeds and almonds) and a banana. One will sustain me until dinnertime, the other will send my blood sugar soaring and then have me crashing and looking for another sugar fix before I know it. Armed with this kind of knowledge, we have power. It is an amazing thing to come to a place where you are not at the mercy of the next chocolate bar or cookie that crosses your path. Give yourself enough time to ask, Is this action going to take me closer to or farther away from my goal? Kelli assures her clients that it gets easier and easier once you understand what each food choice is doing to you and how it affects your body and moods.

Involve your kids

From as early an age as possible, get your kids involved in the kitchen. They can squeeze lemon in and throw the chopped herbs in with the meat. Get them to mix it up with their hands and form little patties to go into the frypan. This is a lifestyle, not a diet. You want to get to a place where you are cooking one meal for all the family, and you need to start developing a family culture that celebrates good food and healthy living. Kids want to copy us and emulate us — whether we are modelling good behaviours or bad. So start showing them healthy habits and great food and their journey towards optimal health in the future will be an easy one.

Think outside the square

The old tuna and salad diet is not something that most of us can adhere to for any length of time. What we need to do is continue to be creative with our eating and look outside the square by adapting recipes and making it fun. When Kelli is approaching a competition and reducing carbohydrates and increasing her protein, she will replace her bread wrap with a large cos lettuce leaf and still enjoy filling it with her flavoursome mince with tomato paste, herbs and seasoning.

Kelli loves bircher muesli where you leave it to soak overnight in milk or water. She soaks the muesli in a little water then adds a *dash* of milk to give it the texture and taste she loves. Over time these little adaptations make the difference between ending up with a body we wrestle with daily or one we can fall in love with each day. You need to look at eating well as a game — balancing good-tasting food with high-energy eating, ensuring you get a little of the good stuff you love, along with a lot of the healthy, fresh food your body needs!

Feelings of deprivation

Number one rule — food should be fun and you should never feel deprived. If you do, that is a sure sign that you are on a *diet* rather than a lifestyle plan that you can maintain for life. What is hard for some of us to understand is that we shouldn't need to eat chocolate every day — if we feel like that, it is a sure sign we are not getting enough rest, or that we are overdosing on sugar and then feeling the blood sugar drop that inevitably follows. We think we need more when really what we need is to feed ourselves properly and get adequate rest. I asked Kelli what she would eat if she felt a real craving for something sugary. 'Protein balls' was her answer, and this is a treat you can now find popping up everywhere from cafés to health stores and even your local supermarket. Or you can make your own by mixing nuts, oats and honey (see Recipe section, p. 201).

Common 'mum' traps

Stop eating the crusts

We can easily underestimate how much food we are getting as a by-product of eating the crusts off our children's sandwiches, or leftover cheese and nibbles throughout the day. This is destructive on so many levels, as we can end up skipping important mealtimes and essentially graze our way through each day eating nothing other than the food the rest of the family doesn't want. We need to prioritise ourselves and get focused on eating five or six small, regular meals every day.

Sit down to eat

So often as mums we rush around the house with a sandwich in one hand, putting toys away with the other or loading the dishwasher. We put multi-tasking ahead of all else in a misguided attempt to get a little more done whilst eating. This kind of mindless eating makes it easy for us to forget exactly what we have or haven't eaten in a day. It can mean we significantly overeat simply because we haven't been conscious of doing it, often just eating out of habit rather than true hunger. Sitting down gives our bodies the signal that it is time to eat, and allows it to process and digest the food in the most efficient way possible — assisting our weight loss efforts if that is our goal, and helping to maintain stable blood sugar levels.

Ditch the dessert

Keep in mind that anything you eat late in the day will surely be stored as fat unless you are able to burn it off. It is the simple *energy in, energy out* calculation. If you are going to devour a king-size bar of chocolate or a large bowl of icecream every night then be prepared for a difficult body battle as the years roll by. A better alternative is to indulge guilt-free in some jelly or a piece of fruit prior to bedtime. For me, the idea of having something after dinner is important — and I confess that for much of the first year of Lili's life that something was as much chocolate as I could consume before falling asleep! Now that I understand what that behaviour was doing to my physiology, and the inevitable mood swings that followed, it is easy to make a different choice. So long as we have some healthy options to hand, this dietary change is pretty simple and achievable for all of us.

CASE STUDY
Antoinette, mum to three girls

Antoinette wanted Kelli's help to change her body shape (to get more curves) and raise her energy levels to help her juggle the demands of her incredibly busy professional and home life.

How old are you and your children?

I am 28 and I have three girls – five, four and two years old.

Were you always very active and health-conscious?

I have always been very active – more so with working and running a business as a personal stylist rather than training. Before having children I would go to the gym one or two days a week and do group fitness classes just for a bit of stress release. I was not as health-conscious before becoming a mum.

Did you have any early role models and what did they teach you?

I never had one particular role model. Like a lot of young girls, I loved movie stars and music stars and all those beautiful girls you see in the media. What this taught me growing up was to strive to look as good as possible, thinking that this in turn would make me feel great on the inside. But that approach can and *did* lead to a lot of heartache for me as I was growing up, as I did not always measure up to the girls in those magazines. But now that I am older and wiser, I realise that we can *all* look fantastic in a magazine if we have been airbrushed and made-over like that! Rather than wanting to look perfect now, like those images, I just appreciate the clothes and make-up that help create the 'look'.

What was the turning point for you that changed your focus?

After having three children my focus was more on wanting to get a better body. I found that my body had changed for the better after having my girls – I felt more 'womanly' and really wanted to see what a focus on training, eating right and not skipping meals could do for me (inside and out).

What about after each pregnancy – did you gain a lot of weight? How did it affect your self-esteem and confidence?

I gained about 15 to 20 kg with each of my children. I did not hold back – I ate what I wanted and didn't exercise when I was pregnant. I was not one of these women who felt beautiful pregnant, and I did not like my pregnant body at all! I did feel very body-conscious and was not confident within myself. If I ever have another baby, I will use the knowledge I have gained from Kelli to eat cleaner and healthier – and definitely exercise!

Was there a particularly low point as a mum? Can you describe how you felt at the time?

There have been lots of highs and lows for me as a mum – definitely with the weight-gain and time-management issues. Making time to train and getting enough 'me time' each week can be tough. At my lowest, I felt very distant from my kids and husband, and not at all happy in my own skin.

What nutritional changes have you made since working with Kelli?

Since working with Kelli my nutrition has done a massive turnaround, not only for me but for my whole family. I now understand the importance of food being the fuel for our bodies and I know how to eat nutritious, easy-to-prepare food. I wanted to *glow* and be radiant and Kelli showed me how to achieve all that with food. I now help my clients look and feel great with these nutrition secrets too!

What does a typical week look like for you in terms of training?

I train with Kelli three to four times a week for one hour or try to fit in Pilates classes as I find this great for core strength and all-over toning. I also go for a run when I can fit it in.

Do you weigh yourself on the scales?

I used to worry about my weight on the scales — as women I think we all do! But now I tend to go more by how I look and fit into my clothes.

What keeps you motivated to continue working out?

I love the energy and the *pumped* feeling you get after you train! I also love being able to maintain my size, and definitely the way I look and feel in my clothes.

What has been the hardest challenge on your health and fitness journey?

There has been two serious challenges so far in my health and fitness journey:
1. My love of all the comfort foods! I love to eat rich and fattening foods, so giving myself the odd 'cheat' day has really helped me to still have my cake and eat it too, so to speak.
2. My self-belief that I can actually achieve my goals, and the idea that I *deserve* to look and feel great about myself … feeling *worthy* of it, I guess. These are things I struggle with at times.

Do you have a support team or system around you to make it easier to fit exercise into your schedule? How do busy mums make time for fitness and health?

Yes, you definitely need support, especially when you have children. My husband and I moved from Sydney to the Sunshine Coast where we have no family to help mind our kids. We rely on each other to alternate minding so we can fit in our fitness programs.

How has your attitude toward your body changed since you were, say, 25?

My attitude towards my body since turning 25 has been a lot more appreciative and I am now learning to love my body. I am actually looking forward to getting older and understanding my body more and becoming that *goddess* that exists inside us all!

Was there a standout moment in which you felt, 'Wow, I'm happy with the way I look!' Have people commented on you being more confident?

My standout moment was my wedding day. I waited a long time because I kept falling pregnant and I really wanted to get married feeling fantastic, which I eventually did! I felt totally amazing physically and mentally, and every time I see a picture or watch our wedding video I am reminded of the confident, beautiful woman I am.

What advice would you give to other women who have recently given birth and are feeling depressed about their bodies?

My advice to other mums is don't start out being so hard on yourself – give yourself enough time to enjoy your baby before committing to your new fitness journey. Also don't listen to women who say, 'I walked out of hospital after giving birth wearing my size 8 jeans!' I totally looked like I was still pregnant when I came home; I then put too much pressure on myself to try to lose my baby weight and didn't stop to enjoy the *experience* of motherhood.

In your job as a stylist, you teach women how to make the most of their shape and body. What should we as mums do to present our best face to the world? A couple of top tips?

A couple of my top tips to start you off:

1. Spend a day getting to know yourself.
Have a good look at your hair, face, nails and body – decide what you need to improve, and acknowledge and appreciate the great features you already have.

The improvements can then be worked on – for example, a new haircut and colour or committing to a personal trainer.
2. Find a stylist (or stylish friend) to help you.
Get them to teach you to do everyday hairstyles as well as the best, most flattering make-up techniques to suit your face and style.

3. Learn about your body shape and have a wardrobe 'dump' day.
Ask your stylist or stylish friend to help you clear out all the wrong clothes and get to work on the *new* you!

Is there anything else you would like to share about your health and fitness journey up to this point in your life?

My theory is that fitness should be something you *love* to do, not something you feel you *have* to do. If gyms and personal trainers aren't your thing, find something that makes you want to get up off the couch, get fit and feel great about yourself.

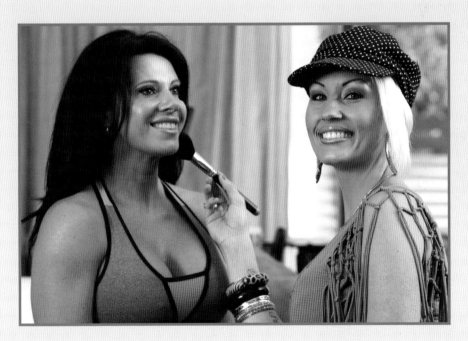

Kelli Johnson with stylist Antoinette Wilkins.

Kelli shares her experience of working with Antoinette

Antoinette is a beautiful young mother of three little girls and was already very slim but wanted to change her body shape and gain a little more muscle. Looking after three children, a husband and her personal-stylist business left very little time for herself, and as a result her nutrition was suffering and her energy levels were very low.

We started by getting Antoinette to eat five smaller meals every day to get the metabolism working again. Then the amount of food at each meal would increase as she became hungry for her meals at three-hourly intervals. This was an indication that her metabolism was beginning to speed up. Initially the food preparation demands were too much for Antoinette, demanding more of her time than she could spare, so I created a meal plan with tasty recipe suggestions that could be cooked in advance to help her keep on top of things.

Being prepared was critical to the success of Antoinette's new eating plan. All the recipes were family-friendly so she didn't feel like she was working in a restaurant dishing out different meals for everyone.

Antoinette would be one of the most immaculately presented women I have ever had the pleasure of meeting – you would think she was happy with everything about herself! Like most of us, she had things that needed improving – she wanted more energy and more curves. We began with three weight-training sessions per week. When we had achieved a certain level of fitness, Antoinette began running, short distances to start with. Once the nutritional issues were sorted out and Antoinette's energy increased, she began running longer distances and then ran with a weight vest on to improve her strength and develop her legs.

Antoinette loves her new shape and the extra energy she now has. She also enjoys training with her husband when she can – there just seems to be no stopping this woman now!

Support

One of the factors we can assume would contribute to our ability to re-establish a fitness routine following pregnancy is support — or more specifically, the level of support we receive.

Only 31% of mums reported that they felt they received enough support from those close to them. Interestingly, mums reported much higher satisfaction levels relating to the support they received from their friends, with 41% reporting that their friends provided adequate support to them as a mum.

The ability to say no

Having the ability to say no implies that a person would have less need of support, as they are less likely to over-commit themselves in the first instance.

Only 10% of respondents indicated that they find it easy to say no, with a further 19% saying they find it 'somewhat easy' to say no. This would indicate that the other 71% of respondents find themselves in situations where they agree to do things that they don't really want to do — this in turn would place additional or unnecessary pressure on their lives. It is possible that this undue pressure could be a factor in our inability to establish or commit to regular exercise.

Older women in our lives

Sixty-three percent of women report having older women in their lives who help them. This relationship could take many forms, including mothers, grandmothers, relatives, older sisters, neighbours and family friends, for example.

This is another significant factor to consider when we begin to look at the reasons women are or are not returning to regular fitness programs following pregnancy. It is worth reflecting on the possibility that we may be being guided by women who, due to their generational circumstances or mindset, are not encouraging or assisting us in establishing a regular exercise routine following childbirth.

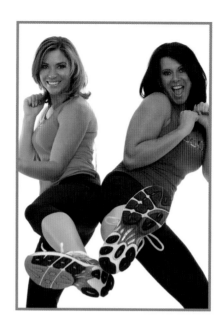

Training

I've learned that everyone wants to live on top of the mountain,
but all the happiness and growth occurs while you're climbing it.

ANDY ROONEY

This next section of the book begins with an important yet often overlooked aspect of any training program for mothers – the pelvic floor. I have asked Australasia's leading pelvic-floor specialist to contribute because I know (from the results of the International Motherhood Study) that over 60% of mothers experience some form of pelvic floor dysfunction post-baby – that's a huge number of us.

Kelli has another top ten training principles for us to embrace, along with some advice for mums just starting out and wanting to get results fast.

So get into your workout gear and put on those sneakers, because after this section I know you will be ready to head for the hills – power-walking or running your way to a sleeker, sexier you in no time!

See you at the top!

Satisfaction with health and fitness

Over two-thirds of the women surveyed reported dissatisfaction with their health and fitness levels (71%).

Only 11% reported feeling satisfied, and just 18% were slightly satisfied. In total, less than one-third of all mothers were satisfied with their level of health and fitness.

Interestingly, almost 80% of those women who *did* feel satisfied with their health and fitness levels exercised on a regular basis (at least three or four times a week).

It is important to highlight the relationship that exists between the high proportion of dissatisfaction with health and fitness, and the low proportion of women exercising regularly following childbirth.

Consult your doctor first

It is important that before you embark on *any* new exercise or nutritional program you consult your doctor and get a clean bill of health. This is especially important if you have recently had a baby or are pregnant as there are many more risks associated with exercising during these times and you need to make sure you are not jeopardising your health or the health of your baby in any way.

Your doctor will be able to help you determine your current level of health and what your ideal weight should be. It's possible that you may be setting goals for yourself that are unrealistic. Acting in response to the covers of magazines touting that it is 'bikini season' is not an effective way to start a health and fitness program. Work with an appropriate health professional and pick a realistic goal to focus on. Don't take off another 2-3 kg just so you can imagine something more unrealistic and harder to achieve — that's a sure-fire way to end up depressed, alone and miserable.

If your doctor says you are at a good weight but you want to be bonier, well, you need to sit down with yourself and really look at what you want to ask of the body you were born with. As we age our bodies change. We can maintain so much of what we are given by exercise and toning and eating right. But we still need to be kind and know that there are limitations. We cannot make our legs longer or put a perfect waist where our body fights against having one. Love yourself … be yourself … and be your best self – not some magazine's interpretation of perfection.

The Pelvic Floor

With author and pelvic-floor physical therapist Mary O'Dwyer

Mary O'Dwyer has over thirty years' clinical experience consulting in women's health. Through Mary I have learnt so much about my own pelvic floor, and also the many ways in which it affects our day-to-day life – including our ability to resume physical activity after childbirth, and our sex lives.

Mary conducts practical and informative workshops for women, helping them to find and control their pelvic floor. Hoping to reach more women than her professional practice would allow, her book *Hold It Sister* (www.holditsister.com) has been designed to transform women's knowledge of their pelvic floor and its important role in the female body.

THE INTERNATIONAL MOTHERHOOD STUDY
Pelvic floor issues

The list below shows the percentages of Australian and New Zealand women who reported experiencing each of the following issues relating to the pelvic floor:

1. Bladder urgency	26%
2. Urine loss with exercise	27%
3. Urine loss with sex	3%
4. Pain with sex	25%
5. Weak orgasm	11%
6. Bowel and wind problems	15%
7. Prolapse	5%

In all, 62% of the 4708 participants in the IMS experienced one or more of the issues listed above.

In addition, 55% of those who were affected did not seek any help or advice.

What is the pelvic floor?

The pelvic floor is the platform of muscles and sphincters that supports and closes your bladder and urethra, vagina and anus. It involves a network of muscles, ligaments and fascia.

Think of this network as a bowl of trampoline-like muscle providing 'lift and hold' for your pelvic organs and closing the sphincters to prevent loss of fluid, wind and solids. Just as a trampoline lifts on recoil, you can draw up these muscles voluntarily, especially during the additional load of sneezing, running or lifting a weight. Pelvic floor muscles should tighten automatically with your deep 'core' abdominal muscles to support your spine and prevent injury while moving.

Guidelines for return to activity following childbirth

Some women recover pelvic floor control at six weeks post-birth, while others may still be struggling with weakness and symptoms of prolapse (where pelvic organs such as the bladder, bowel or uterus 'bulge' down into the vagina) at 12 months.

To ensure the health of your pelvic floor, gradually return to exercise and monitor how your pelvic floor responds to any new activity. Ideally, your pelvic floor muscles should provide good support and control during exercise. If activity forces the muscles down, they will lack strength or coordination and the ability to hold during exercise. The effect of the pregnancy hormone relaxin (which softens your ligaments during pregnancy in preparation for birthing) takes around four months to pass post-delivery.

Focus on postural control and easy walking in the first weeks after delivery and get in shape from the inside out.

The guidelines on the following pages provide a safe framework for returning to physical activity following birthing.

Post-birth return to activity
after an uncomplicated vaginal birth (from *Hold It Sister*, by Mary O'Dwyer)

RETURN TO ACTIVITY
FOLLOWING VAGINAL DELIVERY
For an uncomplicated vaginal birth

E A S Y A C T I V I T Y	24-48 hours	Begin gentle pelvic floor / deep abdominal exercises. Control sitting & standing postures. Avoid Slumping. Catch up on sleep.
	2-4 weeks	Avoid lifting more than baby. Do your PF exercises. Walk 20-30 mins. Have a daily sleep. Seated Fitball balance exercises.
	6-8 weeks	Continue PF strength exercises. Walk 30-45 mins. Daily rest. Basic Pilates & Core exercises.
	10-12 weeks	PF strength exercises. Pool exercises & swimming. Post-natal exercise classes. Walking.
Fitball exercises (NO sit-ups), Tai Chi, Pilates, swimming & pool exercises. Light upper body weights. Graduated return to previous sport. Be aware of PF control.	4-6 months	
Return to light gym: stretch band (sitting and standing), balance classes, Yoga, Pilates, squats and low impact classes. Be aware of PF control.	6-12 months	
Progressively increase exercise intensity & weights (light). Focus on control. Monitor pelvic floor holding strength during all activities.	12-24 months	**I N C R E A S I N G A C T I V I T Y**

This program applies once you have learned the correct pelvic floor
action. If uncertain of what to do, visit a
Women's health physiotherapist.
When returning to gym activities, inform the trainer of your delivery
and any complications during or since.
Listen to your body as it may take 12-18 months to regain your abdominal & pelvic floor strength.

After Caesarean section

The incision made to deliver your baby during a Caesarean section cuts through the layers of abdominal muscle. The sutured muscle layers, connective tissue and skin take time to heal. It is wise to delay your return to activity, and restrict your everyday workload, to ensure healing is uninterrupted.

Recovery tips

- Hold and support the incision line when coughing or changing position.
- Do not lift more than the weight of your baby in the first six weeks. Plan to have help at home.
- As healing progresses, pay daily attention to a 'tall' sitting, standing and walking posture to switch on your pelvic floor and core muscles and retrain your body to the correct posture.
- After two to three weeks, start walking for 20-30 minutes, initially without a pram and avoiding hills. By the end of six to eight weeks, aim to walk for 30-40 minutes, most days of the week.
- At eight to ten weeks, start exercises at the six- to eight-week level for vaginal delivery (see the post-birth return to activity diagram on page 80).

Gym and the pelvic floor

The growth in the number of fitness centres over the last decade or so has had many positives. These facilities promote structured exercise as the 'new way' to fitness for our sedentary society, replacing the incidental exercise that was previously part of our normal work and life activities. Many fitness trends abound, with boot camps, spinning classes, heavy weights classes and intense bursts of exercise. These programs are for the most part too challenging for many women with pelvic floor problems.

Walking, using stairs, gardening, playing with the kids or dancing are proven fat-burners when combined with sensible eating. Slower forms of exercise such as tai chi and yoga, with their emphasis on posture and breathing, make us aware of our bodies' abilities, needs and limitations.

For many gym members the focus is on counting repetitions or minutes rather than awareness of core control. Understanding the limitations of their pelvic floor will empower women to recognise and speak up when a program is too demanding.

If your bladder suddenly becomes urgent or leaks when you sneeze, this indicates a lack of coordinated pelvic floor muscle support. Your gym instructor has absolutely NO idea of your pelvic floor status, and may have little idea about how to avoid aggravating your present problems. They will guide you in all types of exercises without knowing the special needs of your pelvic floor, which is a commonly misunderstood group of poorly trained muscles.

Let your gym instructor know if you have any pelvic floor control problems. If they have your best interests in mind, they will refer you to a women's health physiotherapist and modify your gym program.

If, on the other hand, you have a strong, problem-free pelvic floor, then a gym program should strengthen all the muscles in your body, including your pelvic floor.

Pregnancy, multiple births, menopause and being overweight all put you at greater risk of having or developing pelvic floor problems.

Bladder urgency

An urgent bladder repeatedly sends a signal to empty, making you visit the toilet more frequently to avoid accidents. This can change the way you plan your day, leading you to note the location of every toilet before going shopping, or avoid long trips on public transport. Turning on a tap, putting a key in the door, or heading to the toilet all increase urgency and incontinence.

Important tip

If your need to urinate becomes urgent after exercise, this indicates the level of exercise is too difficult and your pelvic floor muscles are not able to control the internal pressure down onto the bladder. A strong, co-ordinated pelvic floor contracts to counter any downward internal pressure produced by lifting or exercise. Keep improving your pelvic floor control, ask about easier exercise options, and avoid heavier garden tasks.

Red flag questions

Answering 'yes' to one or more of the following questions indicates a need to modify your gym activities and focus on learning the correct pelvic floor and core muscle coordination.

- Do you lose any urine when you cough, sneeze or run?
- Does your bladder become suddenly urgent?
- Does urgency cause your bladder to lose urine?
- Are you currently pregnant?
- Have you had children?
- Were any delivered by Caesarean section?
- Did you experience any pain from pelvic instability during pregnancy?
- Do you have any separation of your tummy muscles?
- Post-birth, did your doctor note any prolapse?
- Have you had any recent lower back pain?
- Have you had any pelvic or spinal surgery?
- Does your mother have a prolapse?
- Do you have any concerns about your bowel control?
- Are you unsure about how to exercise your pelvic floor muscles correctly?

Exercise guidelines for at-risk women

I. Avoid curl-up abdominals and heavy weights

For unfit, post-birth or menopausal women, performing sit-ups, curl-ups, medicine ball rotations, double leg lifts, Fitball crunches or advanced core exercises is the quickest way to promote pelvic floor dysfunction. These abdominal exercises force pressure down onto the pelvic floor, and unless it responds with a quick, co-ordinated and strong lifting contraction, injury is likely.

2. Focus on core control during exercises

Focus on correct posture during all exercises to keep core muscles activated. In response to exercise, the pelvic floor and core muscles must tighten before the abdominals flatten and widen the waist. If the pelvic floor and core muscle control 'let go', stop the exercise and reduce the loading. For example, if you are working out on the leg extension machine, keep your spine tall as you raise and lower the weight. If you cannot hold a tall, strong posture, the load is too high for your core control. Your legs may be strong but your core needs work.

3. Build in relaxation/recovery phases

The pelvic floor muscle endurance required for a long run, a 60-minute interval class (weights, cycle, abs etc.), or a boot camp program is considerable. Ensure the training activity includes opportunities for pelvic floor recovery, to reduce fatigue or allow relaxation from overactivity.

Suitable exercises for at-risk women:

- Pool hydrotherapy
- Seated bike work (for short intervals)
- Treadmill – keep the level flat initially and lengthen through your crown while walking
- Tai chi
- Seated ball balancing with arm movement
- Light arm weights – military press, biceps, triceps, deltoid flies, upright row with postural control
- Lying and seated stretch band exercises
- Four-point kneel, opposite arm/leg holds
- Floor bridging holds
- Basic Pilates mat exercises
- Basic Pilates reformer exercises
- Cool down with a stretching program

As your fitness increases and your pelvic floor control improves, try:

- Increasing repetitions
- Increasing sets
- Increasing resistance loading of weights or bands
- Increasing cardio training time on bike and walker

Focus on learning postural control during exercise, before adding weights. Progress weights slowly and carefully.

Be aware of post-baby blues

Hormonal imbalances post-partum can contribute to incontinence, constipation and post-natal depression. It is normal for ovulation to stop during breastfeeding, leading to lower levels of estrogen in the body. Leaking and loss of vaginal sensation can contribute to depression and may set up negative thinking about the pelvic floor. Mothers with incontinence and sexual dysfunction (loss of libido, urine loss or pain during intercourse, less vaginal sensation and weak orgasm) report an improvement in depression and body image after implementing a pelvic floor muscle training program, as such a program reverses these problems.

Taking action

The book you are holding represents a powerful, holistic tool for increasing your levels of vitality and well-being. What I have attempted to do is provide a foundation of information and understanding to help you understand where you are currently in relation to pelvic floor function. No longer should you accept pelvic floor problems as 'part of being a woman'. I urge anyone who thinks they might be affected by pelvic floor complications to reach out and seek help from one of the many resources available — women's health physiotherapists, childbirth educators and continence organisations.

CASE STUDY

Kate, new mum to Harry

This is Kate's heart-breaking yet all too common story about the frustration of wanting to be fit, healthy and 'whole', whilst battling debilitating pelvic floor dysfunction. Kate's work with specialist Mary O'Dwyer enabled her to move forward slowly towards a life that now includes cardio and resistance training.

Confident, sporty Kate, a 33-year-old psychologist, went from having confidence in her strong and active body to finding she no longer liked or trusted it since the birth of her son, Harry. Kate kept bags with pads and fresh underwear in her car, nappy bag and desk at work to cope with regular accidents.

Forceps assisted Harry's birth after a prolonged second stage of delivery. Kate had previously enjoyed a close, intimate sex life with her husband, but now depression crept in as their relationship was affected by sexual dysfunction. In Kate's words, 'It felt like a switch had flicked off, making everything numb.'

From her psychologist's perspective, Kate wryly noted that if any woman experienced prolonged sleep deprivation, loss of sexual sensation, wet pants and restricted activity (with resultant weight gain), depression was a certain outcome. The turning point for Kate came when she discovered she was not exercising the right muscles. Once she found, controlled and trained her pelvic floor muscles she quickly regained bladder control and orgasmic sensation returned. Her mood became more confident along with her new understanding of her body.

A word from Jodie

I recommend that all women visit Mary's website at www.holditsister.com for further information and resources. Mary's book also provides a more detailed look at every aspect of pelvic floor health should you require more in-depth information. My research work alongside the International Motherhood Study highlighted the seriousness of pelvic floor dysfunction, and after studying the subject further with Mary, I am fully committed to raising awareness of, and destigmatising, this very important issue. It's time we started to talk about it and end the shame, secrecy and isolation that pelvic floor complications perpetuate.

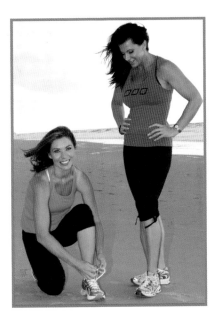

Body Bible Basics:

Training

Ten Success Principles

Keep away from people who try to belittle your ambitions. Small people always do that,
but the really great make you feel that you too, can become great.

MARK TWAIN

I. Develop a plan

As with everything in life, if you don't know *where* you want to go, any road will take you there. Get very clear on what you know you can realistically accomplish. It is important to have both a goal (i.e. to look or feel a certain way) and the *belief* that it is achievable for you. It's all very well wanting to look like a supermodel, but the fact that most of us do not believe we could ever achieve that means if we make it our goal we probably won't even get out of bed when the alarm goes in the morning — it's just too unrealistic. Look around for a role model or inspirational picture that more accurately represents what you want to achieve. I still have a picture taken from a health and fitness magazine years ago. The model looks strong, toned and in control of her body and life. That was the feeling I was after and it continues to inspire me to this day.

Decide what your schedule will allow you to do each day and devise a program to suit. Are you able to train at home or at the gym? Go outside during summer or join a friend in the park? Will it be a morning or evening session? With or without children? There are many factors to consider, especially as the life of a mum is very complex and involves taking into consideration the schedules of so many family members.

Once you have made all the relevant decisions and have a solid plan that you feel is achievable, start making the necessary preparations to ensure you will stay committed to incorporating your program into your daily routine. This might include signing up to your local gym, checking out local bike or running tracks, talking to a friend who might want to join you, or scanning magazines for the one inspirational image that you know will help you stay focused when you have moments of self-doubt or uncertainty.

Motivation boosters

- Get together with a friend or group of friends and support one another in achieving your goals – be accountable!
- Tap into the power of music to motivate you to work longer and harder.
- Don't let the weather be a barrier or excuse – develop alternative options for wet or very hot days, such as walking or running indoors at a gym or using the stairs at your workplace. Think creatively about a solution to ensure you can achieve your goals whatever the weather.
- Keep a training diary to help you monitor your progress and stay on track. Note details of what activity you did, for how long, and how you felt during the day. For further details refer to the Training Journal information on page 105.
- Join a walking or running club in your community – there may even be a mums' group already, or you may like to start one up yourself!
- Have an end goal in mind – perhaps you could participate in a sponsored walk or running event locally. Push yourself to do the work necessary to reach that target. Sign on and pay your registration early, to help you stay connected to what you are working towards. As soon as you complete one event, be sure to decide on another target. That way, your goals continue to push you to the next level.

Try to aim for 3 x resistance training sessions each week (30 minutes using weights or a physio-band at home or at the gym) along with 3-4 cardio sessions (working at a moderate to vigorous intensity for 30+ minutes). You can simplify things by combining your cardio workout and resistance training exercises where possible – this way you reduce the number of sessions required each week to start seeing results. Make sure you give yourself rest and recovery days during the week too.

2. Check with your doctor first

Always get a clean bill of health from your doctor before starting on a new training program. You need to make sure you have no underlying conditions or injuries. If you choose to train with a fitness professional, they will absolutely need to know about your circumstances. You owe it to yourself to get regular health checks regardless of your age. Think of this as an opportunity to check out the health of your physical body, which is after all just a tool to allow you to live your life to the fullest. If there is anything concerning you, make sure you check it out immediately and enjoy the peace of mind that comes from facing your fears rather than allowing them to fester inside and develop into far greater problems in the long term.

TRAINING GUIDELINES BEFORE AND AFTER BABY

Before baby

If you are pregnant you should discuss your proposed exercise plan with your midwife and/or doctor. Take it slowly as your pregnancy progresses, and make sure you are working with an experienced trainer in relation to any gym workout or weight-training program. Walking is the safest and most gentle form of exercise, along with a hydrotherapy program such as an aqua aerobic class. Thankfully there are now many of these classes that are designed specifically for pregnant women, and they offer the additional benefit of being a way to meet other expectant mothers with similar interests.

Gone are the days when being pregnant meant you should do nothing. You can still exercise – just remember you are exercising to maintain a healthy pregnancy, not to lose weight during your pregnancy.

After baby

Depending on whether you had a vaginal or caesarean delivery, the recommendations for getting back into exercise vary. Be sure to read the section relating to exercise and your pelvic floor (see page 80), and make sure you understand it fully. If you have any concerns regarding your state of health, you must talk them through with a doctor.

Continue to take prenatal vitamins if you are breastfeeding, and if you are not, a good vitamin/mineral supplement is advised.

Walking is an excellent form of exercise to begin with, and one you can do with your baby in a buggy. As with other forms of exercise, start slowly and build gradually. An added benefit of exercising outdoors is that it is a proven stress buster and can help clear your mind if things start to get on top of you.

3. Nourish your body

Be sure that you are nourished nutritionally. Both body and mind need to have their nutritional requirements met on a daily basis. You cannot ask yourself to achieve physical change without eating appropriately for your expectations. A good balance of protein, carbohydrates and fats is essential for good performance, weight loss, strength and increased fitness levels. Refer back to the earlier section on nutrition for a full overview of key principles and guidelines.

Water is also critical to hydrate your body during training and throughout the day. Take a water bottle with you whenever you are training. I recommend you buy several water bottles and have them filled up each morning and strategically placed wherever you usually spend time during the day – have one in the car, at work, on the kitchen bench. If you can see it, you will be reminded to drink more and will have the best chance of reaching the required minimum of at least eight to ten glasses each day.

4. Take it slowly

When starting a new fitness program, do not overdo it in the first few days. If you do, it will have a negative effect, leaving you feeling sore and demotivated as it takes you longer to recover. Taking it slowly is certainly easier said than done – most of us tend to start out full of energy and enthusiasm, only to regret that enthusiasm on day two as we are so sore we struggle to sit down on the toilet or perform simple daily tasks!

If you are training in a gym, choose to do a group class or a light full-body workout rather than isolating muscle groups, where you are asking new things of your body. If you choose to exercise outside, start by walking for 20–30 minutes then gradually work your way up to 40, 50 then 60 minutes. If running is more your thing, start power walking and slowly incorporate jogging intervals, then increase the time you spend jogging. Again aim to start with no more than 20–30 minutes each day.

One simple way to monitor your pace and determine intensity level is the talk test: if it's difficult to speak, slow down; if talking is too easy, speed up.

When you start exercising, beginning slowly and increasing the intensity and length of your workout as you go, you will see a noticeable improvement within a week or so. As your stamina improves, the activity will become easier and you will be able to relax into it and actually enjoy physical activity. Before you know it the endorphins will be kicking in, making you feel happier and more energised.

The next step is getting to the point where you feel upset if you don't get to do something active in your day — hard to imagine when you are at the starting gate, but a wonderful place to reach. You realise how great it makes you look and feel, and you really don't want to contemplate a day without doing something physical.

Keep in mind also that rest days are very important for your body, not just to give you some down time but also to allow the muscles in your body time to repair and recover from all the work they are doing. Your progress will actually be faster and your results more visible if you give yourself regular, dedicated rest days and allow your body the recovery time it needs.

Jodie's top tip

The synergistic relationship between nutrition and exercise cannot be overemphasised. If, like me, you have previously tried to diet without any focus on training, you will know how much willpower and hard work it requires. Training without focusing on nutrition can also lead to a negative spiral where you don't see enough results for your efforts to keep up the work required. Combining *both* aspects, as promoted here in the *YSM Body Bible*, is the only way to make this process simple, effective and longlasting — it really is the number-one secret why I feel better about my body now than I ever have in my entire life. How many mums do you know who can honestly say that?

WALKING – A SAFE, EFFECTIVE OPTION

If you have chosen walking as your primary form of activity and exercise, then you have made an excellent first choice. With any form of activity, however, you will find that over time your body becomes accustomed to what it's doing, and it will actually burn fewer calories. There will inevitably come a point where you no longer see the rewarding improvements in your fitness level. This is your signal that you need to shake things up a little.

You need to find ways to continually challenge your body. You can burn off more calories by increasing your speed, or by tackling a steeper incline. To get the most results from your activity time, increase the walking speed on flat terrain. The calorie burn from walking faster on flat terrain is significantly higher than if you just increase the incline (unless the incline is very steep). If you really want to start seeing results then add a little more of both to your fitness regime. Head for the hills and give it all you've got!

5. Start early

Cardio before breakfast is best (after enough sleep and a good dinner the night before). This early activity stimulates your metabolism and starts the fat-burning process. A good power walk first thing in the morning, outside in the sunshine, also helps you to wake up as it slows the production of melatonin (the sleep-regulating hormone), leaving you feeling more awake and energised. You will be ready for a healthy breakfast when you return home.

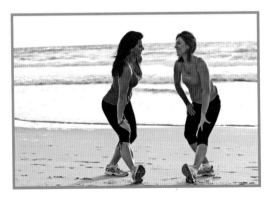

Safety reminders

It can be challenging to stick to an exercise program and schedule regular activity times. Sometimes you may need to get out earlier or later than you would like. By adhering to a few simple safety rules you will be able to achieve a relaxed state and have peace of mind during all your training sessions.

A gym membership is a good option as a way of providing you with a safe place to work out at any time of day, but if this is not possible for you, here are some important safety tips:

· Walk with a friend or family member for pleasure and safety.
· Walk during the day if possible, or on well-lit streets.
· Wear reflective clothing at night.
· Let someone know the route you're taking and approximately how long you will be out.
· Where possible, vary your routes and times so you are not a predictable and easy target.
· It's easier to avoid cars if you can see them coming. If possible, avoid busy roads and those with no footpaths; if there is no footpath, walk on the side of the road facing the traffic.
· Follow your instincts. If you feel that you are entering an unsafe situation, trust your intuition and run to a safe location.

6. Warm up first

The golden rule is always warm up before you train. Damage is done when you ask a cold muscle to do stressful things. If you are weight training, ten minutes on the treadmill or cross-trainer will get things going.

Pain is not gain

Muscle soreness and fatigue ('the burn') may occur with training, and while it's not something that everyone enjoys, it is perfectly harmless. Pain, however, is not. Pain in joints and bones, or pain with movement, should be avoided at all times. You may try to adjust your technique and weight, but if that doesn't work, stop and ask for help.

There is no glory in working through pain, and there will be injuries and perhaps surgery down the track.

Stretching

It is important to take the time to incorporate stretching into your fitness routine. Stretching increases your range of motion and decreases the risk of injuring yourself. It can dramatically decrease your post-workout soreness and stiffness. Stretching in your daily life is also a great way to reduce stress and tension.

Key points to remember:
- Always warm up the body prior to stretching, as this increases blood flow around the body, which in turn makes the muscles more supple.
- After exercise, slowly bring your heart rate down before you begin stretching – this will help you to avoid cramp and dizzy spells.
- Never bounce while you stretch, unless you are doing specific stretches for certain sports, i.e. martial arts.
- Hold the stretch until you feel the muscle loosen off, then repeat for a further 15 seconds.
- While stretching you should feel some slight discomfort; if you don't feel anything, then you may be doing the stretch incorrectly – if you are unsure, ask for guidance from a fitness professional.
- Stop immediately if you feel any severe pain.
- Remember to breathe regularly and rhythmically; do not hold your breath.

7. Know your heart rate training zone

Know your heart rate zones, and stay in the zone. To calculate your training heart rate, first work out your maximum heart rate by subtracting your age from 220.

For example, the maximum heart rate for a 20-year-old is:

220 – 20 = 200 beats per minute

From this you can work out your target heart rate as follows. You simply take your maximum heart rate and multiply it by the percentage you would like to work at. (Kelli recommends starting at around 65%.)

For example, the target heart rate for the example above is:

200 x 65% = 130 beats per minute

Once you know where you should be it is easy to keep in the zone by wearing a heart rate monitor. Although they are not essential, these are very useful devices, and many people find that wearing one helps them keep motivated and focused on their specific training goals.

Frequency, intensity, strength and recovery – understanding what they mean

Frequency

It makes sense that a person who trains three times a week will progress significantly faster than someone who only trains once a week. Put in more and receive more. It's that simple.

Intensity

If Person A and Person B do the same exercise routine for 90 days, but Person A does the workout in 30 minutes and Person B in 90 minutes – their results will be incredibly different. High intensity over a short period of time trumps low intensity over a long period of time. Always. When you are starting out, however, you must allow for rest and recovery periods during each training session. These can become shorter and less frequent as your fitness level improves.

Strength

If we don't push ourselves to get stronger our bodies will have no reason to adapt. This is why some people train for years at the same weight and others achieve amazing progress in only a short period of time.

Recovery

It is with recovery that we grow and regenerate for the next day. Apart from nutrition, your most important method of recovery, weight loss and stress reduction is sleep. An adult should have between seven and nine hours of uninterrupted sleep every night. For many of us mums, that recommendation is far from our reality and completely unrealistic. If you have a baby or are getting up to children in the night, you need to allow for some down-time or rest during the day to compensate.

8. Ask for the help you need

Make sure you feel confident about what you are doing. If you are embarking on a new weight-training program, make sure you know the correct technique for all the exercises. If you are unsure about anything seek the help of a trainer to show you the correct way to perform the exercise. This will help you to avoid injury and make sure you are getting the full benefit of your exercise program.

Weight training is more complex than simply attending a class at your gym. This is where a professional trainer comes in handy. Although they cannot do the actual work for you, they can make your experience more enjoyable, safer and much more rewarding.

Tips for finding the right trainer for you

1. Always check their qualifications. Ask to see their personal training certificates or relevant university degree.
2. Ask them what tools or plan they have to help you achieve your goals. This should consist of a nutritional plan, a tailored exercise program for you to follow and a tracking mechanism to ensure progress towards your goals.
3. Always ask for testimonials. Ideally the trainer should be able to provide you with case studies of past clients with before and after pictures. Perhaps you could speak to another of their clients for reassurance.
4. Ask for a free trial session. Choosing a personal trainer is a big decision and you do not have to sign up with the first one you meet. Try a session with two or three different trainers and pick the one you feel most comfortable with.
5. Look to see if the trainer is 'walking the talk'. Are they a good example of health and fitness? If not, then they probably can't be trusted to motivate and inspire you towards your health and fitness goals.
6. How focused and attentive are they during your first trial session? If they are taking calls from other clients or seem distracted then get out of there! This time should be all about you.

9. Make it achievable for you

Set realistic training goals. Don't expect to run a marathon or compete in a triathlon straight away. External motivation is great but be careful not to place yourself under unnecessary stress. Plan your workouts around the time that is available to you each day. It may not be at the same time each day, but getting out and being active daily is crucial to increasing fitness and health.

Simple and effective cardio options to fit into your day

One of the easiest ways to keep your weight under control is to buy a pedometer and make sure you get at least 10,000 steps in every day. All the steps you do during the day count, and depending on your normal daily activity, you can top up with a morning power walk, a relaxing evening walk or some skipping while you watch the kids ride their bikes.

The bonus is that you know where you are at all times — you have a very clear daily goal, and you get to decide when and how you make up the extra steps you need each day.

Cardio workout 1
Walk a minimum of 10,000 steps in one day (track with a pedometer) or perform a 40-minute power walk before breakfast.

Cardio workout 2
Skip rope for 10 minutes followed by a 20-minute power walk outdoors. Adjust the skipping tempo from fast to slow, to help build-in recovery phases. Increase the intensity as your fitness improves.

Cardio workout 3
Walk, jog or sprint up a hill or large set of stairs as many times as possible in 20 minutes. Finish off with a 20-minute power walk.

Cardio workout 4
Do any cardio-based exercise (rowing, cycling, jogging, swimming) for 30-60 minutes with moderate to vigorous intensity.

10. Continue to set goals

Often we set ourselves a target and reach it only to find we lose all motivation and focus and revert to our old habits, weight or lifestyle. We see it happen to our girlfriends or family members all the time and it can be heartbreaking. What we need to do is continually create a new goalpost so we always have something exciting to work towards.

If it was a wedding day or school reunion that got you motivated to begin with, then once the big day arrives, set yourself another target to work towards so you keep your energy high and your focus on some point in the future. The kinds of goals we are talking about include:

· Competing in a sponsored walk/run in your local community.
· Entering a mini-triathlon event with a few friends — you do the run, swim or bike and they do the other activities!
· Write down a goal to run 5 km or to run for 40 minutes without a rest (that is what Meg did in our case study on page 180).
· Join your local gym and get involved in any competitions they organise for members.
· You might want to compete in a figure championship like Vickie. (See case study details on page 115.)

Whatever it is that excites you, go for it! The only thing that's important is that your goal has meaning for you.

How great to think that you are the only thing that matters in all of this — for once you don't have to make a decision based on the needs and wants of everyone in your family — enjoy being selfish for a change!

Finally, a word on staying motivated and committed to your training

We all have times when for one reason or another our good intentions and focus depart temporarily — leaving us feeling angry or frustrated that we didn't manage to go the whole distance. The secret is not avoiding these times, for they are inevitable. The secret is learning how to handle them, and knowing how to get back into the game as quickly as possible.

Helpful ideas to keep you on track:

1. Allow at least four weeks for results to start showing, and decide to commit to your plan for at least that long. Do everything you can to give yourself a fair chance of

getting through the first few weeks, which are always the most challenging.

2. Vary your program and the setting in which you walk or run. This will keep it fresh and more interesting — helping you avoid burnout and boredom.

3. Walking with a friend or dog will help provide motivation on those days when you are feeling less than enthusiastic.

4. Try not to have an all-or-nothing approach. If you have a tough week, don't beat yourself up — forgive yourself and move on. This is real life and there will always be stuff that crops up to thwart your good intentions.

5. Celebrate success! How can you continually push forward with your goals if you never allow yourself the luxury of revelling in how far you have come? Reward yourself for all the little wins along the way — running for 20 minutes non-stop, or getting to the gym three times each week for a month. Whatever is meaningful to you.

6. Make use of bonus activity every day. That includes things like parking your car further away from your destination and walking; going for a walk during your coffee break; or taking the stairs instead of the lift. Sometimes we can create an additional 30 minutes of activity simply by taking advantage of these small opportunities every day.

7. Be sure to use the time you spend working out to contemplate the great things in your life and the positive things you are working towards. Resist the urge to think about problems like money worries or troubling family issues.

8. You have to do whatever it takes to feel good. Remember, progress can be measured in many ways, such as mood, sleep, self-esteem, weight loss, and energy. The longer you stick with a physical activity program, the more benefits you'll feel.

Keep in mind that of all the things in life that are out of your control, physical activity isn't one of them. Being active is something you control and do solely for yourself. Select activities you really enjoy — swimming, bike riding, dancing, walking — anything you find interesting and entertaining. Team up with a friend, family member or your dog. Whatever you decide to do, be consistent and make it fun!

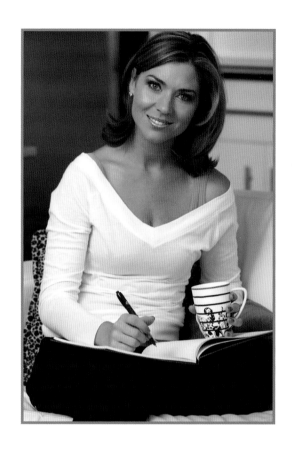

How to measure progress

The way you feel

Keep a written record of how you feel during this transformation and use that as your barometer of success. Include in your diary how you felt each day — your moods and energy levels, along with any compliments you received along the way. This should be all the motivation you need, but if you crave more, here are some additional options ...

Ideas to consider

Before and after photographs

Because you get used to seeing yourself in the mirror each day, it can be difficult to really see the visual improvements you have made to your body. Before and after photos can be a great way to measure progress — especially if you are a visual kind of person. Stick them up on a vision board (see page 223) to keep you motivated as you get closer to reaching your goals.

Remember to:

- Photograph yourself in a relaxed pose from all three angles (front, back, side).
- Do it first thing in the morning on day one or before commencing your new program.
- Include your entire body in the photo.
- Wear as few clothes as possible (it makes it much easier to see the changes).
- Take your before and after shots in the same spot, under the same conditions.

Your clothes

A simple and time-tested method for monitoring progress is to see how your clothes are fitting. Are they feeling looser and more comfortable? Are you wearing things that you haven't been able to wear for a long time? Are your favourite jeans starting to hang off you now?

Although hardly scientific, this method motivates a lot of mums (including me) more than anything else. Just knowing that I can walk into my wardrobe and pick out anything that I feel like wearing on any particular day is success in itself! For too long my life revolved around only being able to wear half the clothes that were hanging in my wardrobe, and I got sick of attaching 'slim' or 'fat' labels to items. I yearned for the day when I would know that I looked and felt great in every single piece of clothing I owned. That is my reality now, and I know it can be yours too!

A note about the scales

The scales are probably the most misleading indicator of success when you follow the guidelines in this book. I totally transformed the shape of my body, dropped a dress size along the way, and received all manner of compliments from people wanting to know my secret, and I did this without even dropping so much as one kilo during the entire time.

Muscle weighs more than fat, so you are actually trying to put on muscle while you lose fat — as a self-confessed 'skinny fat' person I had a lot of muscle to gain, and this countered all the fat I lost in the process. So, don't go buying any scales. Don't get neurotic about what you weigh — it's just a number and it doesn't hold any real power over you. Choose instead to measure your results based on energy levels or the way your clothes look and feel — trust me, you will be so much happier you did!

Body fat percentage

Most people want to lose weight and gain muscle or tone. If you are being successful with your goal of gaining muscle, however, it is possible you may not only maintain your weight, but even gain weight. While you're losing fat, you may gain enough muscle to increase your overall weight. Home scales don't give you this important information — in this situation they would only tell you that you have gained weight, and to most of us this simply translates as bad news. What we really want to know from regular scales, but cannot see, is our body-fat percentage.

The only true way of measuring this is by using body-fat scales. These look like regular scales but they give you much more information, including your fat percentage. Unfortunately quality scales can cost hundreds of dollars, but most gyms have them and if you belong to a gym you could ask to use theirs.

Alternatively you can use skinfold calipers, which is what Kelli uses for her figure competition clients who require a very accurate means of measuring their body-fat percentage each week. Kelli can then adjust their training and nutrition plans accordingly. If you are really concerned with having accurate measurements taken along the way to help motivate you, this is something to consider alongside a fitness professional.

For most of us, our improved energy levels, the compliments we receive and the fact that our clothes fit better will be all the measurement we need — the hardest part for many mums is avoiding the scales, as for so long we have allowed ourselves to feel good or bad based on the numbers they tell us. It can be quite liberating to know that the scales do not provide the answers we need on our new high-energy lifestyle plan.

Try this for a change — throw out the traditional scales and tune in to the way you look and feel each day. That, after all, is the real measure of success in life!

Full blood analysis — an option

This is something you may wish to consider, depending on your personal goals and commitment to pursuing optimal health. Visit your doctor or blood specialist and order a full blood analysis before you begin your new program. This is something you can repeat after two to three months to help track your progress. A blood analysis will show up any deficiencies in your blood resulting from your diet, and can help direct you to the correct supplementation and dietary changes specific to your needs.

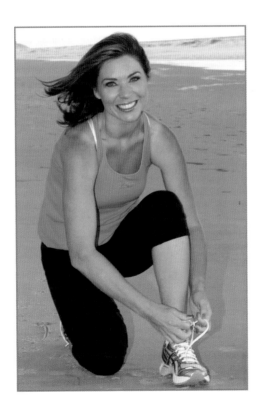

Training planner

This is a tool to help you plan your training so you make sure you have something to aim for each day and week. It also allows you to see where you currently have time to devote to exercise and perhaps where you might need to ask for support to enable you to follow through with your new program.

Try to find five 30-minute training slots within your week to begin with. You can gradually increase this to five 40- to 60-minute training slots as and when you progress. It is essential you allow your body rest days to recover from activity, especially from resistance training with weights.

It actually takes less time than most people imagine to create a body that is toned, lean and strong — brimming with energy and good health. What it does take is a *regular commitment*, and that's where most of us fall down.

If you focus on each day and doing all you can to keep your appointment with you, then the achievement of your goals will be inevitable — not some kind of miracle!

Session	MON	TUE	WED	THUR	FRI	SAT	SUN
Before breakfast			✔		✔		
Morning						✔	
Lunchtime							
Afternoon							
Evening	✔			✔			
Proposed activity: (e.g. running /gym/swimming)	Gym class		Power walk	Gym class	Run	Yoga	

Training journal

This is a simple option to allow you to review your progress and revisit your successes along the way. By checking in daily and weekly to assess the degree to which you are following your nutritional and training guidelines, you give yourself a far greater chance of long-term success. This is not a journal to give you feedback as to your weight or measurements — if you want to do that, then we recommend you do so alongside your doctor or a trained fitness professional. The goal of this journal is to help you stick to the basic principles on a daily basis, and to record improvements in your energy levels, quality of sleep and related factors.

Instructions

Use one sheet for every week and fill in the week number. You can either photocopy the page that follows or create a similar template yourself on the computer.

Put **'Y'** in the **'Nutrition'** box if you followed the nutritional guidelines in this book.
Put **'Y'** in the **'Training'** box if you exercised for a minimum of 30 minutes.
Put **'Y'** in the **'Water'** box if you drank the recommended minimum of 8+ glasses of water.

Be sure to enter your energy level each day, along with the number of hours you slept.

Write down any additional comments that would be useful to look back over as you continue to review and revise your program as you move toward your goals.

It is up to you how specific you want to be within the comments box — what's important is that it makes sense and is motivating to you. You may wish to include information on how you changed your 'self-talk' throughout the day (those voices in your head that love to tell you why you'll never succeed!) or perhaps how you resisted having one too many glasses of wine when out at a social event. Every detail will help you in the future as you build a reference of ideas and strategies that you can come back to again and again.

Additional comments may include information such as:
· Supplements you are taking
· Relaxation or complementary activity — meditation, yoga or sports massage

- Problems you are facing relative to your training goals
- Strategies you discover to assist you with your goals
- Support you received to help you stick to your program
- Unexpected benefits experienced, such as feeling 'less anxious' or 'more tolerant of family members'
- Compliments received.

Training Journal

Week no.

Date:

	Mon	Tue	Wed	Thur	Fri	Sat	Sun
Nutrition Y/N							
Training Y/N							
Water (8+ glasses) Y/N							
Energy level? 1-5 (low to high)							
No. of hours' sleep?							
Additional comments:							

Kelli's workout wisdom for mums

Energy gets energy

Have you ever heard someone declare with absolute and total conviction to anyone who will listen, 'Oh, I'm too tired/busy/exhausted to exercise'? Maybe it was you on occasion (surely not!). Well, those who have read *You Sexy Mother* will know that I have been guilty of that on many occasions, but despite it taking some time, I have finally come to the powerful understanding that 'energy gets energy'.

One of the first things I remember Kelli telling me was this: 'Jodie, there's no way around it. You have to *start* with the exercise and the energy will follow. You can't hang around waiting for the energy to arrive so you can start a fitness program … it will never happen! The exercise is what *creates* the energy you are looking for, and soon you will be able to fit in the exercise more easily and you will start finding you have time and energy to do more things. Who knows where it will lead you?'

Some of us, including me, need to be hit on the head a few times before things really sink in, and that is why there is a lot of repetition of key points throughout this book. This energy thing is a really important concept for you to grasp — we really want you to understand it and we genuinely want you to succeed.

So if you desperately want to tell someone about how your situation is different because you have small children or you don't have any family living close by to help you or you have some health issues that make you more tired than most, then go prop yourself down in front of the nearest mirror and get it all out to the only person who really cares — YOU!

If you are still reading this book you are obviously genuinely committed to creating a positive change in your physical body. You're done with the excuses and really want to learn what kind of mindset you need to join those who look fantastic and feel great in their bodies. Congratulations on getting this far — just think of all the extra time you will have to focus on exercise now that you have decided to stop complaining that you don't have time to do it!

I can assure you there is no better way to generate energy than to exercise — the times when for some reason I have stopped training for a week or two are always the times when things start to get on top of me again. Now that I know the early warning signs, I immediately make a plan to get into the gym or outside for a run and suddenly, as if by magic, my mood improves and so too does the energy in our whole house as everyone once again feeds off Mum's positive energy.

I asked Kelli to share with me some of the key ways in which mums might inadvertently sabotage their success ...

Training too hard, too fast

Kelli has seen this numerous times, where a woman comes in full of excitement and commitment and heads out into the world pushing it all as far as she can go. She runs to exhaustion, lifts weights at the top of her ability and cuts her calories right back at the same time. She also decides to pursue a full-on detox diet and eliminate coffee by going cold turkey. What ends up happening is that her system can't cope with all the sudden changes to her diet and exercise. She experiences pain in her muscles as a result of overtraining without building up the necessary strength first — then finds she can hardly get out of bed the next day. Her headaches are causing her to feel rotten as a result of the caffeine withdrawal, and she feels constantly hungry because she opted for an extreme diet rather than a slow and steady approach that gradually introduces healthier options and portion sizes.

We have probably all been there, and it's so hard because we want to see results fast and we are so eager to get to the finish line. It's no different from our kids wanting to grow up fast because they think it would be more fun to have more freedom. As adults we encourage them to enjoy their childhood and the lessons they learn along the way, and we need to encourage ourselves in much the same way. The results *cannot* be longlasting if you don't learn the lessons along the way — you need to fail sometimes to really learn, and you need to put in the effort to fully understand what it takes to be a person who is committed to health and fitness for life. It might be frustrating and it might take a little longer to get to where you are going, but at least you won't give up after the first week due to muscle fatigue.

Be easy on yourself and see your goal for the long race that it is. There are no medals for heading off faster or going so hard that you stop somewhere on the track. There are only hard-won medals for people who complete the race.

Here are some expert tips from Kel to make sure you are one of those at the finish line.

Who are you doing it for?

Be really, really honest. Is this focus on health and fitness because *you* really want to look and feel your best, or is it because of something or someone else? Is it really because your husband or boyfriend or some girls way back in high school said you needed to lose weight? It's an important distinction, and your answer to this will pretty much determine whether you will make it all the way or not. Kelli assures me that without exception, the one thing that determines which women succeed and which ones fail and drop out is their motivation — who are they doing it for?

If the answer is you, then congratulations, you have an exciting journey ahead! If the real answer is someone else, then put the book down and think of someone else who might benefit from it at this time, because you have some more work to do emotionally before you are ready to start any dietary or fitness changes. You need to do whatever it takes to get to that place where you decide to do something positive just for you.

Ask yourself how would you feel if you made a change? How would you like it if you could fit everything in your wardrobe (or have to buy a whole new wardrobe because everything in it was too big)? If your partner would like to see you looking slimmer and more toned that's well and good, but we are not put here on Earth to provide a pleasing picture for others to look at — anyone can go buy a painting for that. We are here to experience life — to jump, dance, move and feel great. That's the *feeling* place we need you to get to before any of the tools in this amazing little book will work for you. You can get to that place quite easily; it just takes focus — so get focused and let's get moving right along — there's no time to lose! You *deserve* this.

Surround yourself with uplifting, energising support

Kelli showed me the different ways in which she continues to inspire herself after many years as a competitive figure athlete and trainer. She uses everything possible to keep her mind and body positive, including using essential oils, upbeat music, inspirational quotes and learning from others who excel in the field of health and fitness. There is absolutely no reason why anyone cannot do the same things that Kelli does, and here are a few ideas to get you started ...

Essential oils

Do not select the calming, tranquil oils that might be good prior to going to sleep, like lavender. Instead start the day by burning citrus, pine or peppermint for an instant lift. There are many great books you can pick up which share the secrets of how and what to use depending on the effect you are after. Have fun exploring what oils make you feel great and start incorporating them into your life in various ways.

Music

Pick something upbeat that you love to really help you during a cardio session — have you ever tried to run in silence and then experienced the thrill of running twice as far with some great music helping you along the way — it really makes a big difference. When I train at Kelli's home gym, she always puts on music to get us in the mood — yes, it works for romance *and* fitness! Music is such a wonderful way to change your state of mind — it can probably lift you out of the dumps and have you feeling optimistic again more quickly than anything else. This is one tool you can't afford to overlook.

Inspirational quotes, books and photographs

Kelli has her personal vision board proudly displayed in her kitchen, which I think is great. It took me a long time to put my vision board somewhere that everyone who entered my home could see it. I even used to take it down when people came over, and put it straight back up when they had gone. Now I am more open about my goal-setting and sharing this information with others — most of the time people are genuinely interested in what it is and how it works.

Books with quotes or inspirational stories can be very helpful to keep you on track, and Kelli has books as well as photographs around her studio to remind her each day of where she is headed. She even has wonderful pictures of her clients enjoying proud moments looking and feeling great — including a stunning picture of Terri Irwin with her daughter Bindi on the red carpet, glowing and radiating health and vitality. I know that Kelli gets a huge amount of joy through seeing her clients enjoy a positive connection with their bodies, and these photos really help motivate her to continue helping others.

Daily email motivation

Another tool Kelli uses is to sign up for daily inspirational emails via the Internet. Depending on what author you like or what websites inspire you, you could sign up for a daily motivational tip, or a daily inspirational quote — the *You Sexy Mother* community is also a great online group to join if you want to keep inspired in every area of your life and learn what other mums are doing to create *their* best life.

Finally I asked Kelli who trains the trainer? Who keeps Kelli Johnson motivated, inspired and in top shape?

The answer surprised me because it is something all of us can tap into, not just fitness professionals like Kelli. What she does is look at what's happening in the world of fitness internationally. She gets inspired by observing what the top US figure athletes are doing and she enjoys experimenting on herself to see what results each little change to her diet or exercise plan makes. She doesn't have anyone training her on a week-to-week basis; she just soaks up inspiration from all around, and so can we.

Kelli believes that we could all benefit from looking further afield and opening up our minds to the possibilities that exist for us as women. We may not all aspire to be figure competitors or triathletes, but we shouldn't be limited by anything either.

One of Kelli's favourite inspirational quotes is:

The brain simply believes what you tell it most.
And what you tell it about you, it will create. It has no choice.

UNKNOWN

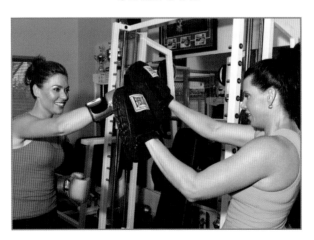

Exercise equipment – what's really needed?

If you've ever thought that getting in shape meant spending hundreds of dollars (if not thousands) on fitness equipment, then you're in for some great news – it doesn't. In fact you don't really need anything other than your naked body and the right head space. Some comfy clothes and a pair of supportive, well-fitted shoes are the next thing on the list, so you can take your workout outdoors or into the gym, and from there it's up to you how much more you want to invest in.

Even if you get everything that's listed below you still won't need a separate room in your house to keep it all in, or a second mortgage on the house – everything recommended in this book is simple, cost-effective and results-driven.

The most important thing to remember is that it is YOU doing the work, YOU getting the results, and YOU that matters – everything else, including the equipment, is secondary.

First steps

If you are just starting your fitness journey and don't have any equipment as yet, the items on this list – particularly the first two – will allow you to do everything outlined in the 'home training program' and get you up and running.

1. Exercise ball (Fitball) – sized correctly for you (55 cm, 65 cm or 75 cm)

An exercise ball, or Fitball as it is commonly known, is a simple tool designed to give you maximum variety and options. It is also a relatively low-cost item that can be stored easily in your home. Not only will your stomach muscles love it, but so too will your kids – just try wrestling it off my three-year-old when he is showing me his 'exerthighzes'! It's also wonderful to use for stretching – after a good workout there is nothing nicer than lying over the ball on your back with your arms outstretched, thinking, Great – that's me done for the day!

2. Set of dumb-bells – either 2 kg, 3 kg, 4 kg or 5 kg

Dumb-bells are incredibly versatile, offering you so many exercise options and taking up very little space. The only tricky part is deciding what weight to purchase in the first place, but you can always ask for some expert help when you visit your local sports shop.

The general rule is not to worry too much about lifting big weights — it's more important that you can do an exercise correctly, because trying to lift a weight that is too heavy will only lead to injuries.

You can always increase the repetitions as you progress, and eventually you might like to own a couple of different sets of dumb-bells — this will help you to perform a variety of exercises and allow you to progress more easily as you get stronger.

3. Exercise band (or physio-band)

To enable you to take your workout on the road during business travel or holidays, the next purchase should be an exercise or physio-band. This is a wonderful item for anyone experiencing pelvic floor dysfunction, and Mary O'Dwyer's book *Hold It Sister* illustrates some wonderful exercises with a band to help strengthen the body without causing any or further damage to the pelvic floor. A band also provides a no-excuses solution for people who lead busy and nomadic lives.

4. Exercise mat

A mat is really a necessary purchase if you are working out at home because it provides cushioning for your spine during your workout and gives you a level of comfort that will make your workout more enjoyable and hopefully have you coming back time and time again. You can make do with a towel over carpet to begin with, but an exercise mat is a simple and cost-effective investment that you will be pleased you made.

5. Medicine ball

Another item you might consider as you progress is a medicine ball — a fantastic little ball that is quite heavy relative to its size and provides you with a variety of exercise options. It is particularly effective for training with a friend as you can do all sorts of throwing and passing exercises to help strengthen your core and work your shoulders and abdominals.

6. Household stairs/park benches

Don't forget the practical 'equipment' around you, like the stairs in your home, which can provide a wonderful cardio warm-up or step-up, step-down platform. The bench at your local park is also perfect for doing step-ups or tricep dips — just start thinking creatively.

Be store-savvy

Just a word of caution when you go to buy things at a sports store. It is their job to sell you products, so don't be misled into thinking you need ten things to be a success in the fitness game — you don't. You just need to take it one step at a time and get the equipment that is right for you. You will need to have an exercise ball that is the correct size for you, and weights that are appropriate for your level of strength, but apart from that it's all pretty simple.

Don't let anyone make you feel intimidated by any of this. It's not complicated and it's not meant to be scary — it's meant to be *fun*. Having a few tools to make your workout more effective, safer and more comfortable is the aim of the day. I don't care where you start, how big you think you are or how unfit you feel — you can do this, and you deserve to be on this road to health and happiness as much as anyone else in the world.

Own your power, do the work necessary, become the best possible you.

I repeat — OWN IT, DO IT, BECOME IT!

Let this be your mantra.

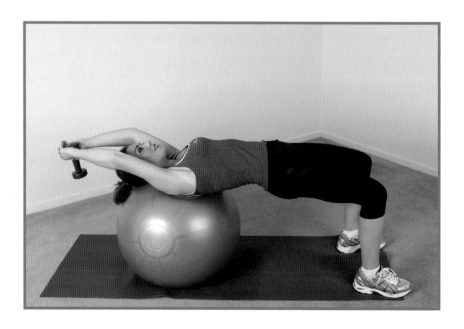

CASE STUDY

Vickie, mum of two young boys

Vickie asked Kelli to help her get back in shape and fulfil her desire to become a figure competitor – after both her pregnancies.

How old are you and your children?

I am 31 and my two beautiful boys are six and almost two years old.

Were you always very active and health-conscious?

When I was in high school I was always very fit – I was involved in a lot of sports and gave everything a go. I found running in my mid-twenties, probably due to the great running tracks in and around Brisbane. I fell in love with the way it made me feel and would go running most days.

Did you have any early role models and what did they teach you?

I really can't remember having anyone special, but I lived in an active household with my mum walking every morning, my dad still playing competitive basketball in his forties, and both my dad and brother being very good basketball players. Many of our social outings were sports-related.

At what age and what stage of motherhood did you decide to train for a figure competition?

I have done two competitions and both times it was about 18 months after having a baby. At my first competition I was 26 and the second I was 31. At 18 months after having each of my boys, I was back in a good fitness routine and was physically ready for the demands of training.

What about after each pregnancy — did you gain a lot of weight? How did it affect your self-esteem and confidence?

I don't know if it was because I was younger but after my first child I bounced back easily and quickly. It could also have been because he wasn't a good sleeper but if I went for a run with him in the buggy he would go to sleep and stay asleep when I got home, so I ran every day. I can't say the same after my second son was born. I had gained a lot of weight during the pregnancy and after he was born I seemed to be always tired and emotional. I didn't really think about my size because I always felt too busy to notice, but I did want to start exercising again and I didn't want my only clothes to be maternity outfits — I kept looking at my previous wardrobe with lust, wanting to wear everything.

Was there a particularly low point as a mum? Can you describe how you felt at the time?

Not so much a low point, but I tried to do a boot camp training session three weeks after having my second child and almost passed out. I felt so frustrated that I couldn't do what I used to be able to do before becoming pregnant. It certainly taught me that I had to listen to my body and start slow, especially second time round.

How did you come to meet and work with Kelli?

After my first pregnancy I kept seeing this very fit, energetic, bubbly woman come in and do her banking where I worked. Before I met Kelli I was keen to do a competition but just never knew how to go about it. So one day I asked her what she did and then asked her if she would train me.

What nutritional changes have you made since working with Kelli?

The nutritional changes I've made are really about knowing what works for my body and knowing that it's okay to eat the treats I love on the odd occasion. I have really embraced the 80/20 rule!

What does a typical week look like for you in terms of training?

An average week of training is an early morning run or swim, depending on my fitness goal at the time. I try to incorporate three weights sessions and some social sports or group training sessions to keep everything fun.

Do you worry about your weight and the scales?

I don't own scales so I can't say I worry about weight! I look more at how my clothes fit as a measure of how I'm doing in terms of weight.

What keeps you motivated to continue working out?

I keep motivated by challenging myself — be it a marathon, competition or by changing what I do and keeping it fun and interesting. I like to run different paths, see different scenery — or try something new like a stand-up paddle-board lesson with friends. I also like going into my wardrobe and not having to worry about whether something will fit or not.

What has been the hardest challenge on your health and fitness journey?

The hardest challenge was during my first competition. The nutrition was difficult as it was very different to what I had been used to eating. The training was hard at times too, especially as I had to do sessions at home and it is so easy to sit in front of the TV instead of working out. Having a goal really helped to get me off the sofa though.

Do you have a support team/system around you to make it easier to fit exercise into your schedule? How do busy mums make time for fitness and health?

I have been so lucky with having an amazing support network around me. I get up early to exercise so I can be home before my partner goes to work, and for my weights sessions I'm fortunate to belong to a gym with amazing crèche hours. The way I find time to fit exercise in is to have a routine and commit to set times during the week.

How has your attitude toward your body changed since you were, say, 25?

I think I'm much more comfortable in my skin now. Before kids I cared a lot more about how people saw me even though I was a bubbly, outgoing person. Since having kids, I am less worried about others' opinions of me and I try to focus on making myself happy. I like to be a goofball as much as I can and just have fun with my kids wherever we are and with whoever is around. I think I'm more relaxed and fun.

What advice would you give to other women who have recently given birth and are feeling depressed about their bodies?

My advice is to take it slow and change just one thing at a time — make it achievable. When you have a setback don't beat yourself up about it; enjoy the break and get back on track the next day, because we've all had one too many slices of cake from time to time.

A very close friend once told me to 'be your own best friend'. Tell yourself what you would tell your best friend if she was in the same position — most of us are always hardest on ourselves. Be supportive of yourself and realise you're not only looking after yourself but also your kids, husband/partner and friends.

Is there anything else you would like to share about your health and fitness journey up to this point in your life?

On reading this I sound like I'm a fitness machine but I can honestly say that's not true. I still have chocolate, fish and chips, pizza — you name it. But now I have those things in moderation. Some days I know I should go for a run or get to the gym but I don't. With the busy life of a mum and looking after a household it's just normal. I don't think I would ever go a week now without doing some kind of activity, but I do think it's okay to sit and take a break sometimes, even away from the pressure of healthy eating and exercise.

Kelli shares her experience of working with Vickie

When Vickie first came to me she told me she had done a lot of running in the past and that she was a vegetarian (absolutely nothing wrong with that). Vickie had a goal of competing in the figure division at a figure and fitness show, so we started out by changing her nutrition and began a vegetarian program supplemented by protein shakes (whey-based). Because of her specific training goals, it was difficult to make the progress she was looking for without more substantial protein foods, such as chicken, fish, red meat and turkey. Vickie decided to incorporate fish and chicken into her meals and this allowed her to build the necessary muscle to help achieve her goals.

There were times of self-doubt and days where motivation was an issue, due to the demands of being a mum with young children and working. Vickie's schedule was demanding and not for the faint-hearted. At one point she was doing an hour of cardio first thing in the morning, before breakfast, every day of the week, along with four weight-training sessions. Please note, this is not your typical training for general fitness and does require consistency and a huge amount of commitment.

We scheduled Vickie's training appointments around her family and work, and she never missed a beat — getting her body into the best shape it could be was a high priority. Not everyone wants to compete at this level but the changes I witnessed in Vickie, both physical and emotional, were amazing. Her perception of herself and her body image went from disapproval to loving herself and her new body.

Not only did Vickie's body transform, but she also had more energy, and improved quality of sleep (requiring less sleep every night). She was eating more food and losing body fat while gaining lean muscle and strength. She developed excellent eating habits that have been passed on to her family, and she no longer feels tired during the day as she is always well-hydrated.

It was wonderful to be a part of Vickie's journey, and she now maintains a well-balanced lifestyle where exercise and good nutrition are an essential part of her everyday focus.

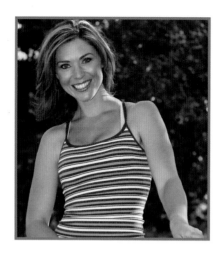

Holistic Well-being

This book was never intended to be something that would add to the already immense and excessive pressure on women to be and get slim. I have spent so many years immersed in the world of plus-size fashion that even the thought of this (to anyone who knows me well) is absurd.

What interests me and what is worth discussing and promoting is the idea of being authentic and in a place of personal power — where we decide what we want our bodies to look and feel like, and where we own the tools and knowledge to make that choice a reality.

I have spent a great deal of time learning the specifics of creating a lean, toned and, most important, vital body. What I didn't anticipate was how much of that journey was going to reside in my head. Until you connect the mind with what is going on in the body, nothing will change for you. Once you begin to understand the interconnectedness of your mind, body and indeed soul, you can then begin to leverage the power of your mind and its amazing ability to assist (or sabotage) you in the pursuit of any goal you might conceive of.

Get ready to begin creating the mindset of a winner. These are the exact steps that elite athletes, successful businesswomen, or effective mums for that matter, need to take in order for their lives to continue in a joyful and successful way.

If you want to know the future, look at what you are doing in this moment.
TIBETAN SAYING

The challenge of change

Change may be a simple six-letter word, but to actually achieve it is anything but simple. There are so many different theories and options available to us, all looking to promote long-term change in our lives. Still the answers seem to elude us and we keep searching for that perfect formula that puts it all into place. Often the hardest, most resistant part of the equation is us! What is required is a willingness to stop focusing on others long enough to truly connect with what we want. What are we *really* looking to change and why?

What are we really looking for?

Often the question of what we want is just too big and scary. We settle for a weak and less than inspiring answer — maybe something along the lines of 'more of the good stuff please'. The truth is that money will never buy happiness and happiness will never pay your mortgage, so abundance in all areas is in fact what we are all striving for. But when it comes to the focus of this book and achieving the goal of feeling good about our bodies, we need to be a little more specific regarding our goals.

Take a closer look

There are three main energies essential to holistic health — your mind, body and soul. They all work together, or against one another, like the currents in a stream. Our strength in each of these different energies will dictate whether we are moving forward, standing still or slowing down, and at what rate. This, I believe, is the real secret to being able to unlock our potential for change.

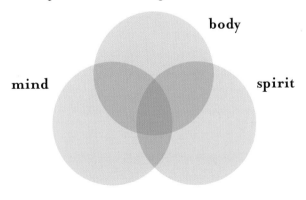

body

mind

spirit

Mind games

*It is confidence in our bodies, minds and spirits that allows us to keep looking
for new adventures, new directions to grow in, and new
lessons to learn — which is what life is all about.*

OPRAH WINFREY

Understanding the power of choice

Take a moment to consider the way in which the choices you have made each day have led to the life you now have and, more importantly, the life you are creating for your future. Remember, your future can be no more wonderful and healthy than the choices you make each day allow it to become.

Unfortunately there will not be a 'makeover mum' fairy arriving at your doorstep to surprise you with a fab new body and exciting life any time soon — you need to be that fairy. You need to start consciously choosing differently so you can create the results in your life that you want.

The diagram on the next page takes you through this simple step-by-step process, so you can see exactly how you arrived at the body/job/relationship/life you have now.

1. We **Choose** (consciously) the way we **Think**
We must Choose with power to overcome any negative Emotional influence.
2. Our **Thoughts** affect what we **Believe**
3. Our **Beliefs** affect how we **Behave**
4. Our **Behaviour** affects our **Result**, **Performance** or **Experience**
5. Our **Result** influences the **Choices** that we make in the future

If the Result is positive, it will create a positive feedback loop influencing our Emotions and the way we Choose to Think. If not, it will create a negative loop.

This is how your past influences your future. The more negative baggage you are carrying around, the more powerful you must be in the way you **Choose** how to **Think**. And the more you do this successfully, the stronger your positive feedback loop will become and the easier it will get.

You are today where your thoughts have brought you;
you will be tomorrow where your thoughts take you.

JAMES ALLEN

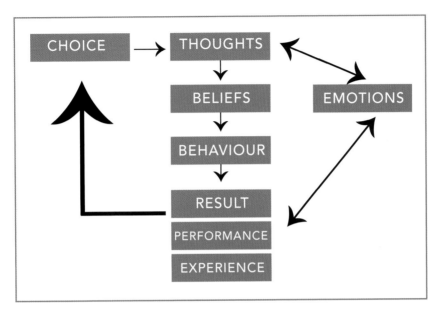

Believe you deserve it!

All that we are is the result of what we have thought.

BUDDHA

Give yourself permission

If you don't permit success to join you on your journey you may find yourself perpetually avoiding it even when it's right in front of you. It may sound stupid, the idea that we have to give ourselves *permission* to succeed in order to do so, but it's not. It is part of our conscious and subconscious self-belief, and without choosing to give ourselves permission we are all in danger of self-sabotage.

You deserve this

You need to believe that you deserve the success that is coming your way. If you don't, life has a funny way of making sure that it won't. A good example would be lottery winners who end up in terrible financial strife after their big winnings, no matter how many millions they had.

Visualise your future

You need to appoint yourself from day one as the rightful receiver of this new body, increased energy, glowing skin and hair. It is important that you vividly imagine yourself having already achieved the changes you are looking to make, revising the image daily and making it clearer every time.

All great achievers have appointed themselves long before they achieved anything. Presidents, athletes, entrepreneurs and other successful figures all believed that they would end up right where they are. It is very rare to stumble upon success, and even when it does happen, we have a unique ability to rid ourselves of it all in the blink of an eye.

Take action

1. Picture a clear mental image of your changed self in the future.
2. Revisit and polish your vision daily.
3. Complete the 'Vivid goal-setting' exercise in the Tool Box section (page 224).

Understand your mind games

There are many mind traps along the road to success ...

The myth of discipline

You are the result of what you love the most. Discipline is merely a reflection of your conviction. Your body will never do anything that your mind doesn't really want to do, because such actions lead to internal conflict and stress. If attempts have gone pear-shaped for you in the past you must change the way you are looking at your goal.

Often people manage to lose weight and shape up for a major life event, such as their wedding day, only to slide back into their old patterns from that moment on.

What they fail to do is reach for a new motivation to keep them striving and creating results in their life. Perhaps a ski-trip booked six months ahead would provide the motivation you need to keep up the momentum and positive change.

Nothing is forbidden

With change there are always sacrifices; some are temporary and some permanent. Your brain can't stand being denied things it knows it really can have (did someone say chocolate?) and so enormous amounts of willpower will be required to stay off the forbidden fruit. What you need to do instead is decide to choose to have something else rather than feel like you are being denied the goodies – the result is the same, but when you make a conscious choice to select or do something healthier, you are the one in control. It will have the same outcome, but it'll use up much less of your mind juice!

The Monday syndrome

Does this sound familiar – life throws a couple of social events your way (along with a few extra cocktails and those hard-to-resist pastry morsels) and puts your health and fitness routine in a spin. So you decide to call the whole thing a complete and utter failure, overindulge some more (because what's the point now?) and start all over again come Monday. This little charade plays out week after week until eventually you shake your head, wondering why it's so hard to move forward with your goals. When this happens we are the ones who are making it so much harder than it needs to be. On an intellectual level we know life will throw stuff at us to send us off-track occasionally – what we need to do is anticipate this and decide beforehand that we will focus on one day at a time and resist the urge to write off an entire week based on one particular day's so-called success or failure.

Remember that two steps forward and one step back will always get your further than one step forward and two steps back.

Emotional eating

If people only ate because they were hungry, this would be a very small book! But instead we eat because we are happy, sad, angry or even bored. Emotions more often than not dictate how, what and when we eat. If there are underlying issues that are causing problems for you, dealing with these will be much more effective than following any eating plan or training program on its own.

Common reasons for non-hungry eating:

· Not giving ourselves enough time to listen to what our body signals are telling us
· Confusing thirst with hunger
· Letting ourselves get too hungry
· Feeling unsure when to stop eating
· Filling up, but not feeling satisfied
· 'Just in case I get hungry later'
· The clock says it's breakfast/lunch/dinnertime: 'mealtime' eating
· Almost any emotion or feeling can trigger non-hungry eating
· Meeting certain needs
· The food tastes great
· Feeling bored or tired
· Worrying that we might offend someone if we don't eat
· Our parents always told us to finish everything on our plates
· We're bombarded with advertising and marketing
· Eating as a reward
· Eating out of habit
· Eating because it's there
· It brings back memories
· Eating quickly
· To solve a problem, fill a gap or put off doing something
· Any combination of the above and many, many more!

Take some time to consider whether your relationship with food is something you can deal with alone or whether you need to take this journey alongside a trained professional. Sometimes we need to work with others to help make the connections that will allow us to move forward in more positive, healthy ways. Don't be afraid to ask for the help you need.

I am most inspired by those who have the courage to reach out for help in life,
as I know first-hand how difficult that can be sometimes.

JODIE HEDLEY-WARD

Endless excuses

Excuses are used to justify our actions to ourselves and to others, and to shift our responsibilities away onto external factors. Conditions for change will never be perfect and thus you will never run out of excuses. It takes courage to take action under imperfect conditions, but doing so will not only bring you closer to your goal but also boost both your confidence and your self-esteem.

Sometimes as mums we can be really great at coming up with excuses that on the face of it sound iron-clad — 'I'm too tired, too busy, don't have anyone to look after the children …' It wasn't until I started training with Kelli that I realised how hollow those excuses really are. Kelli would just look at me and say, 'What, you don't think I'm busy too? I can do it and I'm a mum … and so can you!' She really shone a light on my ability to put up barriers where there weren't any — there would always be a way around it for Kelli. After all, she had spent years working out how to become the best in her field whilst being a mum too.

Kelli knew that excuses would never get her to where she wanted to be, so very early on in her career she adopted a different attitude, that of 'where there's a will, there's a way'. That's the attitude I embraced after meeting Kelli and it has changed my life in so many wonderful ways.

Set yourself up for success

Many people feel as if they have tried to lose weight their entire life, and naturally they want their results to arrive … yesterday! This impatience often results in setting unrealistic goals for ourselves, followed by guilt and discouragement when we fail to achieve the impossible. Science tells us that the average 'quick-fixer' will put the weight back on again plus an additional 15%, while losing muscle and tone in the process. It is a negative spiral that for many has been going on for years, becoming harder and more extreme each time.

Realistic milestones lead to ongoing encouragement that will make the journey much more enjoyable and the end result something that sticks. Get excited about your transformation! Take it steady and make it last.

The need for a spiritual anchor

Happiness is the spiritual experience of living
every minute with love, grace and gratitude.
DENNIS WAITLEY

A common misconception

Being spiritual does not mean that you spend your days in a cave writing down enlightened verses about life, nor is it about going to church every Sunday. The way I see spirituality is like a psychological connection to a higher consciousness or a heightened state of awareness. It's about being aware of something larger than ourselves, and opening our minds to the possibility of there being more to this reality than our senses can tell us — kind of like shades of grey versus a life that is completely black and white.

The missing peace

There is no question that we could all benefit from the inner peace and calm that spirituality can bring, and as busy mothers we often face a tough time trying to carve out the quiet time required to explore this facet of our lives. But as our lives get busier we have more need for going inward to a place of centredness and calm than ever before. Fortunately there are many ways to begin to tap into our inner world and to begin experiencing 'life in the flow'. Start by deciding that you will be open to exploring this aspect of yourself and watch for opportunities that open up for you. Pilates, yoga, meditation or tai chi — these are just a few of the kinds of activities that are designed to help you get in touch with your spirit and experience the beauty of being fully present in your life.

Practise being present

If you are able to sit still for five minutes without letting your mind drift away either to the past or the future, you are way ahead of most people. In the absolute present you are able to experience true bliss and you become untouchable. With enough practice we can learn to escape at times when we really need a break, and also consciously and more effectively control the influence that external events have over our state of mind.

Try setting a goal of five minutes, then see how hard it is to reach 30 seconds. It is harder than you might think! But being able to switch off the past and the future to focus exclusively on the present is an unbelievable tool for any mum, so don't give up — just keep working on it.

There are many books exploring the subject of meditation and relaxation methods, but a simple starting point is just to find a place to sit or lie down, where you won't be disturbed, and close your eyes. Focus either on your breath as you breathe slowly in and out, or on some steady background noise such as a ceiling fan or air conditioning unit. Don't get hung up about the time you spend doing this, just do what you can do, knowing that every minute of deep relaxation is benefiting you greatly.

Explore the possibilities

Open yourself up to the resources available — online, locally in your community and through specialist books. Develop a positive interest outside of your children — something just for you. A spiritual anchor is what we all need to keep sane when life goes into overdrive.

Follow your bliss and the universe will open doors for you where there were only walls.
JOSEPH CAMPBELL

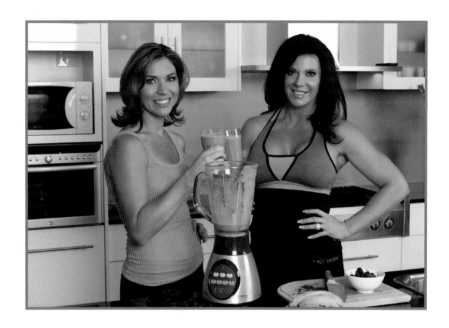

Body Bible Basics:

Setting Up For Success

Ten Success Principles

There isn't a safer place to be in the world than inside our bodies when we feel great about ourselves.
DR ANGELA HUNTSMAN

Always be ready to have the time of your life.
UNKNOWN

1. Take the first step

Sounds pretty easy, doesn't it? Then why do so many of us start out the New Year with a list of wonderful goals and high expectations, only to feel like failures after realising at some point in the year that we didn't even take the first step towards achieving most of what was on that list?

Motivation's great — it's pretty easy and cheap to get your fix — but finding a compelling enough reason to follow through with the plans that made you excited to begin with is the real secret. You need to get enough juice flowing, enough adrenalin — your heart rate needs to soar as you contemplate life as it would be if you achieved your goals and started living your dreams.

There are two simple questions to ask yourself in relation to each of your goals:

1. What will I miss out on in life if I don't achieve this?
2. How will I feel if I do achieve this?

Let's be honest, there's no point in setting aside ten precious hours a week to finish your degree in accounting if you feel absolutely no joy around the idea of being an accountant. If you are only doing it to make other people feel good (yes, I am talking about your parents) or because you think you will gain more respect and admiration from others, then it just isn't going to happen for you. Don't waste another moment of your one shot at life walking this empty and meaningless path — this is a clear example of what actually happens when women say, 'I tried to lose weight/get fit/study/*fill in the blank*, but it was just too much for me and I had to let it go.'

That's nonsense — we let it go because it never excited us enough in the first place. I bet you know of someone (maybe that someone is you) who found the time, willpower and motivation to get fit and healthy prior to their wedding. Or maybe you know of someone who after a financially difficult period in their life started to really excel in their chosen career. These people had what I call hunger for success. At a very deep level they associated not achieving their particular goal with a lot of sadness, disappointment and missed opportunity. They also associated the achievement of their goal with a huge positive shift in their current situation.

Sometimes being comfortable is a dangerous place to be. You never want to get so comfortable that you get complacent. Sometimes the best place to be is rock-bottom. *You Sexy Mother* was born out of my unhappiness with where my life was at. Emotionally, physically and spiritually, it was a difficult time, and if you put in all those raw emotions and mix it up with a little faith and a clear vision, you have a powerful pill that can propel you to wherever you want to go in life.

Throughout the world there are so many examples of people who have risen from nothing and achieved greatness. It doesn't matter if your goal is to be able to run around the block without stopping or to become a competitive sportswoman — we can all be comforted by the fact that if things do not feel good for you right now, it's okay. In fact it might just be the best thing ever to happen to you, if you allow it to push you past the pain into a place where you are willing to do what it takes to create change. What a gift our emotions are — try viewing painful emotions as simply the necessary trigger in life to show us it's time to take action.

Sometimes the hardest step is the first. When I started this journey, working on increasing my energy levels and overall health, the first couple of weeks were extremely challenging. There were so many opportunities to say, 'Stop! I don't want to do this any more.' Luckily, there was something inside me quietly encouraging me to give it one more day, to implement one more positive change.

Often we get so caught up in the fear of failure that it stops us dead in our tracks. We worry what might happen if we announce our plan to the world and then don't follow through. My approach is to say, 'So what if I fail — what's the worst that can happen? I can always go back to being the way I am now.' One particular week my goal was to write 6000 words, which is pretty ambitious considering I only work part-time and like everyone else I have a lot of other projects going on. I ended up writing just over 4000 words. I probably could have beaten myself up about it and used it as a good excuse to show that I would never meet my publishing deadline, so why bother? I suppose I did have the 'mum' excuse to pull out if I had wanted.

What I did instead was congratulate myself on the 4000 words I did write! I made an effort — I showed up, so to speak. So, the week didn't play out as perfectly as my schedule on the computer — life just isn't like that. Meetings went on longer than expected, family members needed special attention, and on one occasion I just didn't feel 'plugged-in' to writing, so I went and did some exercise instead. Is that failing? It depends on who's doing the judging, and luckily for you — it's you!

Keep in mind the idea that *you* are the one that matters in all of this. Yes, obviously we care what our children, partner, friends and family think too, but when it comes down to it most people are so busy living their own lives that they haven't got time to worry about you. You must make *yourself* proud first and foremost. You must make yourself happy. You need to be able to look at yourself in the mirror in the days, weeks and years to come and feel good about who is looking back at you. Not in a vanity sense, but in a deep, soulful sense. How would it feel to truly like the person you see there — to want to be her friend, to have her as a mother or significant life partner? You need to start making decisions relating to your goals on the basis of whether those goals are taking you towards the person you ultimately want to become.

They say that achieving your goal is not the ultimate reward, but attaining the character and life experiences to *enable* you to achieve it is. There is a very powerful difference. If we relate this to exercise and nutrition, it's the same as saying becoming slim, strong and fit is secondary to having the wisdom, discipline and knowledge to maintain that desirable state.

Before we can achieve anything in life we need to be excited about it. We need to feel intense joy and anticipation as we imagine what life would be like, but we also need to remember to jump in and make that start. Stop worrying about what might go wrong, and start vividly imagining it going right.

No one achieves great success without experiencing failure along the way – the only true failure in life is the failure to participate and give it a go!

> *I haven't a clue how my story will end, but that's all right.*
> *When you set out on a journey and night covers the road,*
> *that's when you discover the stars.*
> NANCY WILLARD

2. Be intentional

I believe this is a critical yet underrated secret to success in any area of your life. I want to encourage you to be very 'present' as you go about your day. So often we find ourselves reaching for a packet of crisps or a couple of cookies or munching on our children's leftover snacks out of nothing more than mindlessness. Often we are unaware how much the 'little bit here and little bit there' is actually contributing to the body we have and are so desperate to change.

It wasn't until we had a guest come to stay with us for a few weeks when Josh was a baby that I became conscious of how much I was actually snacking in addition to my main meals. This young girl was studying nutrition and was on her way to becoming a personal trainer. One day I asked her what I could do to improve my eating, which I believed at that time was quite healthy. She was hesitant at first, trying not to offend me too much, but went on to say she had noticed how often I would eat a slice of cheese here or half an avocado there, whilst preparing meals for the kids. I argued that these were both healthy foods, and while she agreed she pointed out that they were also relatively high in fat — although great when consumed as part of a healthy meal and in moderation, they were not such a great choice for snacks when my goal at that time was to slim down and tone up.

Sometimes we are not ready to hear the truth, but that little insight really stuck with me. I started to monitor how many times I would snack during the day, and it did surprise me. It was like I was consuming another main meal without so much as a thought or a moment's pause to enjoy the food. I decided that perhaps it *was* actually possible to prepare food for my family without taste-testing every component of their meal at the same time.

We can all be guilty of racing about and rushing through our activities so much that we don't give more than a fleeting thought to what, when and where we are going to eat. What I can tell you from experience is that you need to change the way you think about food. It needs to become very important to you, and something you do plan for and consequently really enjoy. It's not good enough to put ourselves last all the time, relying on scraps and leftovers to meet our most basic nutritional requirements.

We are searching for *optimal* health within this book, not mere survival. And if we want to look and feel our best, we need to be fully aware of all our food-related activities, starting right now. The good news is, you will be rewarded with a body that works efficiently and happily towards all the goals you set for it — a friend rather than an enemy on your life journey. What a gift that is!

3. Be prepared

Two little words that will make or break your ultimate success — be prepared. This is true for so many areas of your life, but none more so than your health and fitness. If you don't plan for success by scheduling exercise times each week and preparing healthy food options the night before, your fanciful imaginings of a healthier, sexier you will remain just that — a dream, there in your imagination but perpetually out of reach.

But it doesn't have to be that way. The first week or two will be the most challenging as everything feels a little awkward and you have to think really hard to make it all happen. But luckily, after that it gets easier and easier. Your healthy changes and new food choices will start to feel natural and less contrived. Your fridge and pantry will start to reflect back to you the food choices you know you should be making, and the new friends you meet each time you make the effort to exercise at the gym or in the neighbourhood will start to inspire you to get out more and more often.

A little preparation in the beginning will take you a long way when it comes to your results. You can follow the plan a little and you will see *some* positive changes, or you can take it to the next level and get serious about your results. Make the choice to get proactive and work hard to prepare the night before to ensure you are following the plan on a much more spectacular level, and guess what — your results will be pretty spectacular too!

I encourage you to re-read 'Kelli's kitchen tips and tricks' (page 63) for all the inspiration you need to achieve real results. Kelli has made preparation into an artform. She doesn't listen to excuses (she's heard them all a million times) and she won't be fooled by someone saying how busy or tired they are. She exemplifies the other side of the coin to the saying 'Failures don't plan to fail, they fail to plan' (in the words of Harvey MacKay, the best-selling author and motivational speaker) and as a result her success in sculpting an internationally applauded physique has improved as she has aged — how many of us can say the same?

I always secretly wondered whether it was actually possible to get my best body yet post-motherhood, and since working with Kelli I do feel my body is better than it ever was before, certainly in relation to what matters to me — it's stronger, more toned and brimming with energy. I can honestly credit Kelli's 'be prepared' approach to life for much of my personal success. I make sure that before my head hits the pillow each night I have done all I can to make the next morning run smoothly.

That includes putting my sneakers and running clothes beside my bed so I have to literally trip over them every morning when I get up. This was one of Kelli's first suggestions, and as you can imagine, it works. I don't bother with make-up or fancy hair, I just focus on getting those clothes on and heading outdoors or to the gym as soon as possible, before my self-talk gets the better of me. Usually by the time I have listened to the end of the first song on my iPod I am in a good head-space and ready to give it all I've got.

I have enjoyed life a lot more by saying yes than saying no.
RICHARD BRANSON

4. Think yourself slim

When we change the way we look at things, the things we look at change.
DR WAYNE W. DYER

Stay with me for a moment, because I don't want you to think I have gone too far with this outlandish claim. I admit it does sound a little corny and every bit too good to be true, but I am not the only one who subscribes to this theory.

On about week four of my 12-week program with Kelli I experienced my first week of being tempted one too many times and having to attend one too many social functions in a short space of time. This had interrupted my training plans and well and truly pushed the limits of my 80/20 healthy eating focus. I contemplated the idea of making some pathetic excuse about why I couldn't come and see Kelli that week to be weighed and measured within an inch of my life, but instead I decided to take the high road and just tough it out and be honest.

'Kelli,' I began, 'it's been a tough week, and I have let myself down on both the training and the eating fronts, to be honest.' After encouraging me not to beat up on myself and instead start moving on, Kelli began the standard series of tests. Then she looked at me in amazement and said, 'Jodie, your results for this week are impressive. You have had a major increase in muscle mass and your body-fat ratio is significantly improved – well done!' After wiping the astonished (and yes, delighted) smile off my face, I asked Kelli what she thought was going on here. I confessed once again how poorly I felt I had performed that week, and asked her how it could be possible to have such a great result despite this.

'I think you basically "thought" yourself slim,' she said matter-of-factly. She went on to tell me that she has clients who because of their mental attitude seem to attract weight to themselves like honey to a bee. Then there are the clients like me who have a strong desire to change their relationship with their body and who mentally prepare for success well before they see any actual results. 'When a client embraces success mentally, that's when I know we are going to see results, almost regardless of actual physical effort,' Kelli went on. There is a secret, almost unspoken component of success that in many cases seems to determine our fate, and that is our mental attitude.

So I will leave you with this thought – are you today mentally preparing yourself to win or lose the body battle? Take the time to get your head aligned with the idea of success and your results will surely follow. The journey toward success will probably be much smoother, and infinitely more enjoyable as well. What a waste of precious energy, to be battling constantly with the idea that we might not ever succeed. Far better to accept the inevitability of your triumphant success, and work away steadily towards its sure and certain arrival.

We can think ourselves thin and we can think ourselves fat — mostly the battle is won or lost in our minds.

5. Eliminate stress

For fast-acting relief, try slowing down.
LILY TOMLIN

We respond to all stress through a system designed to keep us alive in dangerous situations, commonly referred to as the 'fight-or-flight' response. In the modern world, even though our lives are rarely threatened, there is plenty of stimulus. This means we are in an extended state of stress, which gives our bodies little chance to recover and takes an enormous toll of our systems. The way this plays out in our lives includes the following less than wonderful outcomes:

1. Sex drive/libido may decrease significantly.
Result: Stress affects your hormones, reducing your levels of testosterone and your sex drive.
2. Abdominal fat stores may increase.
Result: This is directly linked to greater health risks and a not so attractive-looking mid-section — eek!
3. Metabolism may slow down.
Result: You burn less energy, which makes weight-gain easier and weight-loss harder.
4. Cravings for more fatty, salty and sugary foods may increase.
Result: You become more prone to making unhealthy food choices.
5. Blood sugar levels may become altered.
Result: Mood swings, low energy levels and difficulties burning stored fat.
6. Blood pressure may increase.
Result: Potentially serious health implications related to heart disease and stroke.

CORTISOL, THE STRESS HORMONE

The hormone cortisol is produced in response to stress.

Cortisol is important for many of our bodily functions, including regulating blood sugar levels and blood pressure, providing energy for activity, and assisting with general immunity and healing processes. Whenever our bodies are stressed, either physically or emotionally, they respond by secreting cortisol.

Cortisol is responsible for fat and carbohydrate metabolism, providing fast energy during the fight-or-flight response. What happens in the course of our lives as mothers, however, is that any stress, such as emotional stress in response to our children or feeling overwhelmed, creates the same stress response but without the expenditure of much energy. Our appetites increase and the only result is an expanding waistline over time.

Stress, therefore, is more than just an inconvenience or an annoyance; it is something very serious that we need to work at eliminating if we are ever to commit seriously to a healthy lifestyle in the long term. Any efforts towards stress reduction will be rewarded with a biochemistry that is working for you, rather than against you, in your efforts to achieve a leaner, healthier body.

This stress literally creates walls around your ability to lose weight. Think about it.

According to your body, there is a real threat to your life, so why on earth would it waste your precious fat reserves in what may be a time of need?

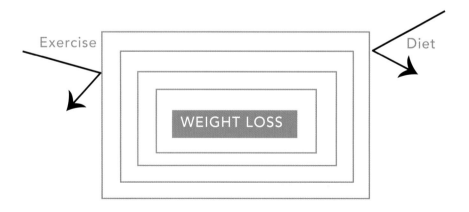

Stress: you have two options

There are really only two ways you can remove stress from your life. Taking no action or the wrong action will only amplify your stress levels.

1. Eliminate

Let's say your stressor was time-related; decide to take action to change the situation. If it's true that you are always doing a thousand things at once, make a decision to eliminate some of your commitments and practise saying the word 'No'. Nothing is so important that you should choose it over your health; if you think it is, you need to seriously evaluate your priorities.

2. Accept and deflect

Not all stressors can be eliminated, at least not immediately. Your next best option is to 'accept and deflect'. This means that you accept the presence of the issue but choose not to react in a stressful way. This can often be applied when we consider family members or, dare I say it, the in-laws.

An example might be that you feel stress whenever your in-laws come to stay for holidays or family celebrations. Perhaps you feel judged, or the situation heightens any insecurities you may have as a mother, wife or homemaker (and trust me, you are not alone in this). To accept and deflect the stress, you might continue to invite your in-laws for holidays, but rather than allow yourself to become stressed and tense, you might work out with your partner that you will go to the gym each day during their stay, to ensure you have the necessary time-out and also to recharge and enjoy the adrenalin buzz that floods your body after exercise.

Take action

· List and prioritise your biggest stressors in the order in which they affect your life.
· Create a plan to eliminate the stress or to accept and deflect it.
· Use one or more of the following stress-reducing techniques daily.

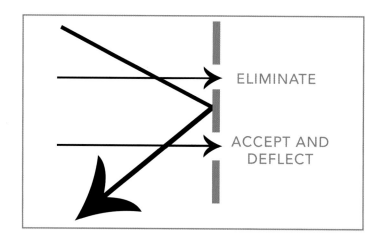

Ten stress-relieving techniques

How beautiful it is to do nothing, and then to rest afterward.
SPANISH PROVERB

1. Breathing exercises

Sit, stand or lie down in a relaxed position. Slowly inhale through your nose while counting to five in your head, then exhale through your mouth while counting to eight. Do this five to ten times to relieve tension, or for several minutes as a form of meditation.

2. Physical exercise

Hang in there for at least 20 minutes, after which your body will release endorphins, which makes you feel happy.

3. Listening

Shutting your eyes and focusing on every single sound you can hear is a good way to shift your attention and allow yourself to relax. This is also a great technique if you find it hard to fall asleep. Just open up your bedroom window, close your eyes and pay attention. It sure beats counting sheep!

4. Guided relaxation

Listening to a guided visualisation and progressive muscle relaxation exercise can be a great way to cope with stress. If taking a nap is not your thing but you know you need more rest or relaxation, this can be an excellent, relatively quick option to fit into your day. Use it when you go to bed at night to help switch off, especially on those nights when your mind starts working overtime trying to solve the problems of the world.

5. Time management
Take five to ten minutes (with a cup of calming chamomile tea) and write down your most critical tasks for the day. Once you have them all down, give them a timeframe (10 minutes, 30 minutes, 45 minutes) and prioritise them according to importance. Usually the tasks you put off are the ones you really should be finishing first. Try this for a week and see if time management could be the answer to drastically reducing your stress.

6. Sex
Having sex is one of the best stress and tension reducers there are. It's fun, it's free and most of the time, our husbands and partners are only too happy to oblige. What's more, it burns calories and helps sculpt a great body (if you do it enough). What's not to love?

7. Playing music
Choose music that gives you a really positive feel with a slow to medium tempo. Avoid music that is too fast or frenetic as it may have the opposite effect.

8. Meditation
When you meditate, your brain enters an area of functioning that is similar to sleep, but with added benefits you can't achieve any other way, including the release of certain health-promoting hormones. Learning to mentally focus on nothingness keeps your mind from working overtime and increasing your stress levels.

9. Vitamins and antioxidants
A multivitamin and antioxidant supplement can successfully cover your deficiencies not only in stress-related vitamins, but the entire spectrum that your body requires. Seek advice from your doctor and/or health professional.

10. Sleep
Sleep truly is a wonderful thing – keep reading for more information on the power of sleep.

SLEEP

We all know that sleep is important, and when you become a mum everyone tells you that you need to rest when baby rests and to take time for yourself — the hard part is actually following that advice as there is always something important that requires your attention and thwarts your efforts to get the rest you desire.

Well, what if I told you that lack of sleep can actually hinder your ability to lose weight?

It appears that eating well and exercising are only two-thirds of the answer to getting and maintaining the body you want. The third, lesser-known component, which is apparently equally important, is something many mums crave — sleep!

Increasingly, researchers around the world are finding that a strong link exists between sleep and the hormones that influence our eating behaviour. There are two specific hormones at work and this is how they can sabotage even the most motivated mum:

Ghrelin   is the hormone responsible for feelings of hunger.

Leptin   is the hormone responsible for feelings of satiety — it effectively tells our bodies we're full and that it's time to stop eating.

Here's the important part — when you are sleep-deprived (99% of new mums take note) your ghrelin levels increase at the same time as your leptin levels decrease. Talk about a double whammy for us wannabe sexy mothers! Not only does sleep deprivation increase our appetites, but it also reduces our ability to feel full. This results in increased cravings that are very difficult to satisfy.

Add the fact that sleep-deprived people tend to choose different foods to snack on — mainly high-calorie sweet, salty and starchy foods — and it's not too hard to see why we end up resenting or avoiding every mirror that crosses our path.

OPTIMAL SLEEP FOR WEIGHT LOSS

Most of us need between seven and nine hours' sleep each night – some more, some less. But how many of us actually get the minimum of seven hours? Motherhood gives us many blessings, but sleep, at least in the early days, is not one of them. Many of us rise much earlier than we would otherwise choose to if it were not for the little people in our lives. If you are pregnant or have a baby, you probably won't remember the last time you got a full seven hours of uninterrupted sleep.

So are we doomed never to be able to lose weight while getting up to our children through the night? Thankfully not. Luckily we can help counteract the hormonal effects of prolonged sleep deprivation. We can work at resting while our baby rests during the day, or at the very least enjoy some down-time where we relax with a book or just sit down during the day. Anything is better than running ourselves ragged all day long and continually pushing our bodies to perform on just a few hours' sleep.

One thing is clear: when your body is not hungry for sleep, it won't be so hungry for food either. That should be all the motivation you need to grab a book and hop into bed for an early night whenever possible.

Joyce Walsleben, author of *A Woman's Guide to Sleep*, says our bodies' hormones have a 24-hour rhythm. 'When you disrupt sleep, you disrupt your hormones,' she says. 'You become glucose intolerant, you want to eat more, and you don't metabolise what you eat as well.' This hormonal disruption can lead not only to weight gain, but also to an increased risk of developing diabetes.

Key reasons (besides children!), according to Walsleben, for disrupted or poor-quality sleep include:

1. Stress or anxiety
2. Noise
3. Light
4. An over-committed schedule
5. Caffeine
6. Alcohol
7. Stimulant medications
8. Depression or anger
9. Fear

Sleep strategies to consider:

It is important to ritualise our cues for good sleep (just as we do for our children — bath, stories, bed), using the bedroom only for sleep and sex. It is not a home office and/or storage room for items that no longer fit elsewhere!

Relax. On the left-hand side of a notebook list all the things that are running through your mind, and on the right-hand side list actions you can take to help resolve those issues. If you are worried about money, write that on the left. On the right list options to ease the situation, such as postpone a holiday, cut up your credit cards or stop buying takeaways. Get those thoughts out of your head and allow your mind to switch off for the night.

Resist temptation. Alcohol, caffeine and high-sugar snacks can all interfere with your ability to sleep soundly. Try to substitute healthier, calmer alternatives such as chamomile tea before bed.

The good news is that exercise will help you fall asleep faster and sleep longer than if you don't exercise. It will also increase your endorphins — your brain's feel-good chemicals, so you'll be better able to deal with stress. Good news for mums and our children!

THE INTERNATIONAL MOTHERHOOD STUDY

Sleep

The general sleep recommendations as outlined within this book range between seven and nine hours of uninterrupted sleep each night. In the IMS a significant group of women fell well short of those recommendations, with over a third of the mothers (36%) reporting that they slept just six hours or less on average each night, and 10% reporting they slept just five hours on average each night.

Although almost 60% of women are managing seven or eight hours' sleep a night, only a lucky 5% get the full nine hours!

Sleep deprivation is known to affect key hormones that in turn can affect a person's ability to lose weight. These statistics indicate that 36% of the women who responded fall into an at-risk category where you would expect their sleep habits to be interfering with their hormone balance and their ability to maintain a healthy body weight.

6. Conduct a self-audit

Life is just a mirror, and what you see out there, you must first see inside of you.
WALLY 'FAMOUS' AMOS

Why self-audit?

By auditing yourself you become aware of your strengths and weaknesses. This is a fantastic tool to allow yourself to break through some limiting belief patterns and negative behaviours. Use it to avoid or alter situations that until now have compromised your success, and to develop opportunities for personal growth. You can make your audit broad or targeted to a specific area — it's up to you.

I need help!

If you find it difficult to be objective or if you have an easier time listing your strengths than your weaknesses (or vice versa), get some friends to help. For accurate insights you want to use only your five to ten closest friends, and just to be sure they won't be too polite to tell you the truth, make it anonymous. In this digital world you could also have everyone email their results to one friend in the group who puts it all together and emails it to you. Why not do it as a group exercise, then everyone can help each other at the same time.

What opportunities am I looking for?

Basically you are looking for strategies to counteract or improve your areas of weakness. If, for example, a weakness is that you always buy fast food on your way home from work, opportunities may include taking an alternate route home or never leaving work hungry. Perhaps you could use the money you save to buy something more enjoyable and healthy, such as a massage at the end of each month.

Take action

- Use the Self-audit sheet that follows as a guide.
- Write down all the strengths and weaknesses that you can think of.
- Write down opportunities based on strategies to counteract or improve your areas of weakness. You may have several for each.
- Put your strategies into place and tick them off as they are successfully executed.

Self-audit (Health & Fitness)

Strengths

Weaknesses

Opportunities / strategies

7. Set your goals

*Winners take time to relish their work, knowing that scaling the mountain
is what makes the view from the top so exhilarating.*
DENNIS WAITLEY

Create goals that are durable, vibrant, clear and realistic

If you are going to achieve anything in life, you need to have a goal to strive for. It needs
to be long-term, specific and above all inspirational. It obviously needs to be realistic,
but also exciting enough that you want to do the work required to get there – this is a
delicate balance to get right. Beyond that, your goals need to change as you change.

Establish an emotional connection

Emotions affect our behaviour more than we think. Our emotional or limbic system (as
it is also called) greatly influences our actions but on a subconscious level. This system
does not understand logic, therefore it is much harder to influence it consciously. If you
really want to ace your goal-setting, then you *must* follow these steps.

With each goal you need to find that *emotional connection* that makes achieving it matter.
This differs for everyone, but you may find your emotional bond in the answers to the
following questions:

· How has my life been affected by not reaching this goal?
· How would my life look if I did reach this goal?
· What possibilities would open up to me in life as a result of achieving it?
· How would I feel if I had this right now?

You may also find your connection by mentally visualising yourself having achieved your
goal, and making the picture as colourful, warm, clear and vibrant as you possibly can.
You need to make your image represent the very experience of being where you want to
be – where you need to be.

Find a visual representation of your goal

Go through magazines or search the Internet looking for inspiration. Cut out or print
a high-quality copy of the image that embodies the result, the feeling or the experience
that you are looking for. Have fun with this – set aside an evening or some quiet time

to really get into it, perhaps doing it alongside your partner or a group of like-minded friends.

Take action

- Use the 'Vivid goal-setting' sheet as a guide
- Write down your champion goal
- Describe the emotional connection
- Find your perfect visualisation and glue it to your 'Vivid goal-setting' sheet
- Look at it daily and practise imagining yourself achieving your goal
- If your goal changes or is achieved, create a new sheet and start again

Vivid goal-setting

Champion goal

Emotional connection

Inspirational image/representation

8. Prioritise self-care

Self-care is not selfish — it's essential.

KIM MORRISON & FLEUR WHELLIGAN

My book *You Sexy Mother* was dedicated to the idea that we should celebrate ourselves in the here and now — not when we are slimmer, prettier, having a good-hair day or have the perfect relationship. I encouraged mums to reconnect with themselves and rediscover their passions in life. I also wrote about the need to start taking better care of ourselves.

A vital component of any training program is rest and relaxation. But rest alone is not enough. We need to take the extra step of nurturing ourselves and giving ourselves the love, attention and pat on the back we all need on a regular basis.

Recently I was being interviewed for a 'Happiness' feature for *Marie Claire* magazine and the contributing editor asked me why it is so difficult for mums to find the 'joy of motherhood' in those first few months and years. I explained that motherhood actually gives us an important gift — ironically, through surviving an extended period of time on minimal sleep, with the words 'I don't matter any more' scribbled all over us!

Motherhood gives us the first real opportunity in our lives to discover things that make us happy from within, things that have no external meaning. We are finally free to explore a life of simple and authentic joy, without relying on the crutch of a compliment, a word of praise or a job promotion, as presented to us by the outside world.

Most mums don't have a team of people patting them on the back each day or telling them how vital they are to the success of things. I was lucky enough to have a husband who would tell me I was a good mum, and parents who tried their best to make me feel that this job really mattered, but so many mums don't even have that. So what we do is try our best to find happiness within our role as mothers, and we can do that in some very different and sometimes bizarre ways — anything from drinking too much in a bid to unwind at night, to becoming overzealous domestic goddesses attempting to keep our homes looking like something out of *Vogue Living* magazine.

We can't see it at the time, but we are trying to recreate the work environment we came from, where we worked hard and in return received validation, approval and status. All we receive as new mums at home are numerous opportunities to perfect the art of the nappy change and how to get the groceries done at lightning speed so we can be at home before the inevitable meltdown presents itself.

What I discovered during this time of early motherhood is that I get a huge amount of joy from only having things that we truly need, use and enjoy in our home. I consciously downsized our belongings, gave excess paraphernalia away to friends and charity shops, and streamlined our lives so I felt more at peace and life felt simpler. I also learnt that being in the water gave me a huge amount of pleasure – just floating and playing about with the kids whenever we could. Before motherhood, I had never had even the slightest connection with the water, apart from taking swimming lessons as a child and knowing I could hold my own from a survival perspective.

My fondness for creating spaces revealed itself – whether it meant building a cubby house for the kids or a special sanctuary just for me where I could curl up by a window and read a magazine while I had a cup of tea when I needed to. Just small, undiscovered, simple joys that I don't think I would have accessed if it had not been for the onset of motherhood and the enforced seclusion that you experience when you are at home with a totally dependent little being for those first few months and years.

So when we talk about self-care, we don't necessarily mean the movie-star options, like booking a week's holiday in the Hayman Islands, or being able to indulge in an all-day beauty spa session each month. Yes, I think that would be heaven, but it is not necessary – and that is the point. Joy comes from so many sources, and if we let money, time or distance from health retreats be barriers to our enjoying some 'me time', then we are allowing something external to be our excuse for not enjoying life to the full.

One of my favourite things to do in all the world is to spend a couple of hours op-shopping, fossicking for vintage finds and handed-down treasures that I can personalise and call my own for less than the cost of a takeaway meal. Read more here …

If there are any other secret op-shopping aficionados out there, eagerly moving from one Salvation Army op shop to the next charity store, then welcome! There is something so seductive about having an hour or so to search for the perfect one-off scarf, dress or worn-once designer shoes that have for one reason or another found their way to the charity shop. I find it so relaxing, and the thrill of the chase is very addictive!

My friend Angela and I have pledged that no matter what the state of our bank accounts, we will always continue to enjoy our love of op shopping together. I have worn my vintage finds to many a You Sexy Mother *gathering and even the odd television interview or two. Some of my most complimented outfits consist of great finds picked up around the op shops here on the Sunshine Coast.*

Just the other day I found a gorgeous black dress (brand new with tags) and realised that it was the same dress I had tried on just months earlier in a shop but (with all the willpower I could muster) decided I didn't need and had left it hanging. Here it was for just $8.95, calling out to me and reinforcing my belief that it's not the clothes so much as the hunt that gives us pleasure. Hunting for treasures at the op shop means I can still indulge, but it won't get me into trouble with my credit card down the line. It also feels good to be giving my money to a group of people in the community that I know really appreciate it and will use it well.

So whether you enjoy op shopping, painting or reading, take ownership of your own well-being and do whatever is necessary or indeed possible, according to your unique set of circumstances. Do anything, just don't neglect the most important person in all of this — you!

You are absolutely, 100%, no good to anyone else unless you take care of YOU. You are so important to so many other people, and you must never underestimate the power you have to influence the lives of those you love. Your children, and your partner if you have one, all feed off you for energy, joy and love. In order to give, you need to receive first. You need to be full so you can give out whenever necessary and still have plenty in the tank to keep going.

You are so important. So worthy. So loved. Remember this always.

*It is always wise to stop wishing for things long enough to enjoy
the fragrance of those now flowering.*
PAT CLAFFORD

*I find myself wondering sometimes if I am the only mum who feels bad about feeling bad ...
how crazy is that? Beating myself up for feeling sad, angry or resentful about some
crisis in my own life — worried that compared to others, I still have nothing
serious enough going on to warrant feeling this way.*
EXTRACT FROM JODIE'S DIARY

Self-care

When it came to asking women if they felt they were good to themselves, just 14% strongly agreed that they were. A further 28% agreed slightly that they were good to themselves, but the majority (58%) did not feel that they were good to themselves.

Alongside this trend was the low percentage of women who responded that they get the 'alone time' they need on a regular basis. Only 13% felt that they did get the alone time they needed, with 18% reporting that they did 'somewhat'. On the other hand, 35% of women strongly disagreed with the statement, and overall 69% did not feel that they got the alone time they needed on a regular basis.

Almost two-thirds of the mothers who agreed that they got the alone time they needed also agreed that they were good to themselves. A strong positive relationship was shown between getting the alone time we need as mums and reporting that we feel we are good to ourselves.

A similar result was found when we asked mums if they were able to 'find time to do activities they enjoy regularly'. Just 18% agreed that they did find time, and a further 21% agreed 'slightly' that they found the time. Over half the mothers did not find time to do activities they enjoy regularly.

There are many factors associated with issues of self-care, such as access to a support network, self-confidence issues and the ability of these mums to say no to external pressures, and these will be explored in due course.

Be nice, for everyone that you meet is fighting a harder battle.
ANITA RODDICK

Here I am,
Where I ought to be.
LOUISE ERDRICH

9. Embrace your emotions

The work will wait while you show the child the rainbow,
but the rainbow won't wait while you finish the work.

PAT CLAFFORD

I learnt a long time ago that we shouldn't devalue our feelings. Emotions are all relative — your pain at being made redundant or losing out on a much anticipated opportunity is no less valid than someone who has experienced the loss of a loved one or received a serious health diagnosis. We need to give ourselves permission to experience the full spectrum of pain and sadness, and indeed grieving, regardless of the socially acceptable version of its perceived seriousness.

Our emotions are complex, and most of us can relate to the idea that events can affect us differently according to other circumstances or things that are taking place at the time — so we may be able to deal with a health or relationship crisis when everything else is humming along nicely, but it would potentially send any one of us over the edge if the same situation arose following the birth of a child or after relocating overseas where we no longer have a strong support network. The context, not just the event, is equally (if not more) important in determining how we will cope in the ensuing days and months.

Your success with regard to your health and fitness goals will improve, and be more profound, if you fully acknowledge and allow your feelings to come through and be felt. Now that you have adopted a clean, healthy approach to your life, you are no longer allowing sugar and refined foods to mask your emotions and falsely 'protect' you. You probably *will* feel more exposed, more vulnerable, more scared … and it's okay. It means you are on the path to becoming a free, authentic, *real* woman who expresses all aspects of herself openly and without fear of judgement. Your ability to then deal with all the emotions that arise will ultimately be what sets you apart and inspires in other women the courage to do the same.

It is more powerful than you think to live your truth — to release the *mask* of motherhood. Free yourself and inspire others to do the same!

HORMONES AND WEIGHT GAIN

Hormones are often talked about in a very negative way — as being the reason for many of the different health issues we are faced with. Actually, hormones themselves are not the problem, and in fact they play an important role as messengers in our bodies. They travel in the bloodstream and direct the functioning of the brain, kidneys, liver, respiratory and nervous systems.

When our hormones get out of balance, however, we start to see complications and visible changes in weight. Below are the key hormones that impact on our weight.

Estrogen

Estrogen is produced in the ovaries in females. A decline in the levels of estrogen directly results in weight gain as the body works to get the necessary amount of estrogen from other sources. Our fat cells produce estrogen; therefore our body will convert calories into fat in order to raise estrogen levels. Unlike muscle cells, however, the fat cells do not burn many calories and the increased amount of fat in your body makes you look and feel 'bulky'. This process is especially common around menopause.

Progesterone

This hormone is also produced by the ovaries, and it declines during menopause. Progesterone leads indirectly to weight gain because when levels are low, the body tends to retain water in its cells. This is known as bloating, and the water retention gives the appearance of being heavier.

Testosterone

Testosterone is necessary for building and maintaining muscle. Any fall in testosterone levels results in the loss of the body's muscle mass and a slowing down of the metabolism, which leads inevitably to weight gain. During menopause our testosterone levels decline more rapidly.

Your body needs hormones to carry out its functions, but any rise or decline in hormonal levels can affect it significantly. The most obvious result is often the gaining of weight — therefore a focus on gaining adequate sleep, eating nutritious foods and exercising will assist you greatly.

Prescription drugs

It is important to note that the oral contraceptive pill and hormone replacement therapy (HRT) contain synthetic hormone substitutes that are not natural to your body and will further disrupt your hormone balance. Talk through any issues you may have with your doctor to ensure you are making the right choices for your body.

Other drugs that can cause weight gain are steroids, nonsteroidal anti-inflammatory drugs (NSAIDs), antidepressants and diabetic medications.

10. Synergy

Just remember, none of these things work in isolation. The reason so many people at your gym are working out every day but are still not satisfied with how they look is because they don't understand the power of nutrition. It's the same reason why so many slender people do not look particularly fit and healthy — they don't understand the importance of incorporating resistance training and cardio into their weekly routine.

Here's the bottom line, girls — nobody can look like Heidi Klum, Jennifer Aniston or anyone else you can think of who looks great on the red carpet without integrating good nutrition and exercise into their daily life — it just won't happen.

It's all terribly simple at the end of the day, and to think it took me 33 years to learn and absorb all this is sad. But I'm so pleased it didn't take me any longer, and I don't want even one mum out there to waste another moment of her life thinking that this thing she has going on with her body has to stay that way.

So this synergy message is short and sweet — get it straight that nutrition alone will not work (at best you will only end up as a skinny fat person). Exercise alone will not work for most of us, and even if it does, you will be making the process far harder than it needs to be. It takes both these things along with a good dollop of sleep, patience, self-love and perseverance.

Whip that lot up and you *will* have created a gorgeous vision that makes you smile with pride when you look in the mirror — pride that you did it, pride that you finally 'got it', and pride that you went the distance.

When you have that moment, please remember to email me, because I want to hear every delicious detail of how that moment feels. For me the feeling was more than words can describe — and when you're a writer that's saying something!

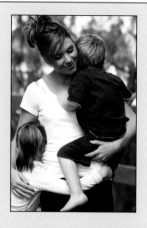

CASE STUDY

Jodie Hedley-Ward

**Read what Jodie shared with _Cleo_ magazine in an
interview about 'Your body after baby'**

How old were when you gave birth? How many children do you have?

I was 27 when I had Lili and 30 when I had Josh.

**When you fell pregnant, did you anticipate the dramatic effect it would
have on your body, even after the birth?**

I don't think anything can really prepare you for the full effect that pregnancy
and childbirth has on you — physically, emotionally and otherwise. I was
prepared for the weight gain and I embraced my full belly during both
pregnancies — ecstatic that I no longer had to hold my stomach in when wearing
fitting clothes. I still think a fit, healthy body with a full, rounded, pregnant
belly is one of the most beautiful things on earth. I'm probably crazy but there
are days when I almost miss my 'bump'. It was like carrying around a little
friend wherever you went — somehow you never felt like you were alone. A very
comforting thought during those countless trips to the toilet in the night!

How exactly did the pregnancy affect your body?

I stayed reasonably fit throughout my pregnancies simply by walking whenever and wherever I could. The weight around my middle was hard to shift post-birth and there was a distinct period of time where all I would dream about was fitting back into a cool pair of jeans – I splashed out on a great pair of Diesel jeans as soon as I was able to do them up. I ended up having two emergency caesareans, so my lower stomach was a very tender and vulnerable area for me for a long time – especially after the first operation.

How did the baby weight affect your lifestyle at the time? Would you do things to hide your body?

This extract from my book *You Sexy Mother* probably sums it up best. We moved from New Zealand to Australia's Sunshine Coast in 2007 (where we knew no one) with a baby and toddler, and this is how I felt ...

During a particularly hot summer, I found myself drowning in despair as every time we went to the beach I would be dressed inappropriately, desperately trying to cover up all the bits of me I wasn't happy with. Instead of frolicking wild and free, dressed in shorts or a bikini as I would have liked, I was covered up with so many layers that I looked set for the shopping mall, not a carefree day at the beach. I felt embarrassment, anger and despair – something had to change. It was time to create a body that was strong, healthy and glowing – one that reflected the way I felt about my life on the inside. I didn't want to waste another precious day feeling inadequate in any way. I didn't want the body of a model, I just wanted the best body that I could have – perhaps even the best body I had ever had!

How did it affect your self-perception?

For me, not being able to wear the clothes I wanted really affected my self-esteem and confidence. I did a thesis at university for my Master of Business degree on the plus-size fashion industry. I had never been plus-size myself but was always passionate about the idea of all women (regardless of size) being able to find clothes that fitted and that made them look and feel fabulous. Now it was my turn to feel less than ideal about my weight and I really understood how these women felt and how weight and body image can attack us deep within — to the very core of our soul — affecting almost every decision we make.

Was there a particularly low period? Can you describe how you felt at the time?

I think my lowest point was when for a very short time I bought into the idea that 'this is it'. The idea that it wouldn't get any better, and that my best body, indeed my best years, were behind me. Luckily I am an eternal optimist and that didn't last long. Instead I set out to prove that motherhood can act as the catalyst for creating your best life ever and that it is possible to get your best body ever. Perhaps not the body of an 18-year-old, but the best body you are capable of having. I am now living my dream life — combining motherhood with writing and researching and feeling better about myself and my body than I ever have. I know it is possible and it is possible for us all — not just a chosen few.

What was it that made you become less self-conscious? Was there a turning point for you, in deciding that you had to change your outlook?

I began to write my book *You Sexy Mother* after a vivid dream one night, one in which everything in my life was very small and shrinking fast. The dream woke me up to the fact that my life was becoming very comfortable and I was retreating to a small world of non-adventure and humdrum. I decided the very next day to change every aspect of my life and start pursuing the life of my dreams.

Who helped you come to terms with the change and grow comfortable with your body? Did you join any support groups?

The first key thing I did was to join a gym with crèche facilities. That gave me a chance to have some much-needed time out from my daughter and the opportunity to rebuild muscle as well as increase cardio fitness and energy levels. I asked for support from my husband and family to make sure I could prioritise exercise each day — I knew instinctively that I could never live the life I truly wanted until I increased my energy levels.

What sort of things did you do to get healthier and feel better about your body image?

I stopped eating the kids' leftovers and actually prioritised my own nutrition. I went from eating a meal here and there, to six small, regular meals that included protein in each. I started to drink loads of water each day and embraced some kind of daily exercise. Not rocket science, but it works like magic!

Are there false ideas (e.g. as perpetuated by celebrities) about how quickly people can lose baby weight?

There is a huge amount of pressure to lose baby weight these days, and the celebrities with their team of experts do make it look incredibly easy. I think there comes a point where we just have to focus on our own authentic journey towards well-being — investing as much energy as possible in making healthy choices each day that will inevitably lead to the body we desire.

How has your attitude/view toward your body changed since you were, say, 25?

I feel more grateful for my body now and I also feel more in control of my body. Pregnancy woke me up to the amazing ability of our bodies to change and adapt and I used that knowledge to help me reach my health and fitness goals.

I love the muscles I see in my arms, knowing that they are the result of lifting my beautiful children up for loads of cuddles throughout each day. I have even made friends with the huge scar on my stomach because it reminds me that two amazing children made it safely into this world.

Was there a stand-out moment in which you felt, 'Wow, I'm happy with the way I look!' Have people commented on you being more confident?

Stand-out moment? No, it just sort of evolved. My journey has been slow and steady and now I am in a very good place.

People do comment about how fit I am now, but they mostly comment on my energy level and the way I seem to do so much but don't appear to be stressed or complain about anything. Now that I work out most days and eat a very healthy diet, I can fit so much more into life. I have a wardrobe full of clothes that fit (that has to be one of the best benefits of eating well and working out). Shopping is fun again!

What advice would you give to other women who have recently given birth and are feeling depressed about their bodies?

Keep in mind that 'hearing the word "mummy" is a gift not a given', and get out for a walk in the fresh air with baby each day. Sunshine is like a magic elixir, lifting moods and giving us energy. Show your baby the raindrops on the leaves and the butterflies in the breeze and just be. And remember always that 'this too will pass'.

How do busy mums make time for fitness and health?

They have to realise that exercise gives you energy — it never takes anything away. The bottom line is, we don't have time not to exercise!

OPPORTUNITIES ARE EVERYWHERE

Once you get into the swing of it, you will start seeing opportunities for activity everywhere – doing squats in the kitchen while you wait for dinner to cook, or walking lunges down the driveway to check the mailbox. It doesn't have to be a big deal – you don't have to think you've failed if you don't get to the gym for a full hour, five days a week.

Sometimes I get out for a run around the house for 15 minutes before my husband leaves for work and I still feel proud of myself – I know that every minute counts and 15 minutes today means I will probably do something again tomorrow. It's the small things every day or done regularly that count, not the 60-minute 'perfect' training session that never happens – that kind of thinking will only doom you to failure because you just can't keep it up.

Body hatred

Having worked with and interviewed many fuller-figured women during my years in the fashion industry, I feel like I have a pretty good insight into body hatred and body dysmorphia. I recall once getting angry with a colleague who walked into our office at the fashion company I worked at and announced to the room that she was 'so fat and felt disgusting'. She was probably a size 10-12 and her comments made me sick to the stomach as there were women in our office much larger than her and I knew in my heart what her comment was doing to their sense of self-esteem.

I took her aside and asked her to imagine how the other women in the room must have felt when they heard her comment, to which she replied, 'I've never thought about it like that.' Her self-loathing comments are commonplace in every school, workplace and social setting you can imagine. What we need to be mindful of is that our comments, even those directed toward ourselves, have a ripple effect that is larger than we can imagine. The best thing we can do is not to monitor where or how loudly we voice our hatred of our bodies, but instead work on changing our relationship with our physicality and move to a place of self-love and self-respect.

This is an issue I am very passionate about as I know how widespread and detrimental our negative self-talk and thoughts can be. Rather than improving over the years, things have escalated, and our self-loathing has reached epic heights in response to all manner of images coming at us from magazines, television, the Internet and billboards.

This book is not about achieving some uniform 'ideal standard' or stressing you out any more than you already are. It is about reconnecting with your physical body in a positive way. Understanding that you are a spirit in a physical body and that it is all interconnected. You cannot feel good about yourself if you don't feel good in your body. Equally true, you cannot feel good about your body (no matter what the size) until you feel good about who you are on the inside — it is all connected in a perfectly inexplicable way.

Clinical psychologist Dr Angela Huntsman shares with us her interesting perspective on the body hatred issue:

We do something quite destructive to ourselves. We tell ourselves and others that we 'hate our body'. Wow, we *hate* our body. What a message to send to a living, breathing miracle of cells that make up one of the most amazing machines ever seen on the face of the earth. So let's break this down. Do you hate your body? Did your body wake up and hatch a plan to get fat or unfit without you knowing about it? Did your body create a secret mouth that it feeds without you knowing? Ridiculous isn't it? Yet why isn't it ridiculous that we can actually hate our body when it only reflects how we care for it?

Shall we become really honest and authentic with ourselves and actually come to the realisation that what we really hate is how we have treated and cared for our body?

Do you really *hate* your body?

Love the fact that your body and mind are full of life; choose to be healthy and happy. If you have had children then you know that from the day we are born and the nine months before that, life is nothing short of a series of miracles. The healing process of a simple paper cut before your very eyes is no less special or beautiful than a camera capturing a flower blooming. Can you see that to mistreat your body is to leave your riches in life on the table?

So what should we do? Love your body. Apologise to it. It looks exactly the way you have been treating it. You ought to hate the way you *treat* your body if in fact that is what you have done. It was made for adventure — running, jumping, climbing, walking, playing — and what do we do instead? Sit around because we feel too tired.

Heroes and hardship

Think of someone you admire — chances are they had to overcome a hardship of some kind. What hardships do you have? Use them to make you stronger. Does obesity run in your family? Use that as a hardship to make you stronger in your fight to keep your weight to a healthy place.

We know more about genetics than ever before — and we are learning some striking facts. How we live has a lot to do with our genes. A life lived well with thoughtful care to the things that matter may never switch on that cancer gene that runs in the family.

My message is simple — you hold the power. Think about your body in terms of how you are treating it, not whether it is *good* or *bad*. Refuse to spend another moment hating your body, or anything in your life that is within your control to change.

Take your power back using the tools and strategies from within this book — you have everything you need to create a brand new reality for yourself, starting today!

Have you ever been to a party and noticed that oftentimes it isn't the most beautiful person that is the most attractive to others? Being engaging and attractive comes from within. Don't use becoming thinner or fitter as some sort of personality fix. You won't become more 'attractive' if you come closer to some sort of visual ideal you set for yourself. Work on the inside separately.

DR ANGELA HUNTSMAN

Changes in body image and satisfaction with appearance

Just 7% of women reported that they felt better about their body since having children, and only an additional 11% reported feeling somewhat better about their body since having children. This leaves an overwhelming majority (82%) who don't feel better about their body after children.

We can safely conclude that body image is a significant issue post-baby for the women who participated in the study.

Furthermore, only 12% of the women reported being satisfied with the way they look, with only a further 21% feeling 'slightly satisfied' with their appearance.

This means that two-thirds of mothers are not satisfied with the way they look.

However, just over one-third of the mothers who reported they were not satisfied with the way they looked agreed that they felt their husband or partner found them attractive, while over three-quarters of those mothers who did feel satisfied with the way they look felt their partners did also find them attractive.

Also, 40% agreed that the way they felt about their body impacts upon their desire to be intimate. This percentage grew to two-thirds of the sample (over 3000 women) when we included those who 'slightly agreed' that their feelings about their body affected their desire to be intimate.

These numbers highlight the flow-on effect of how a woman's self-perception can impact on her partner or husband. **Even at this preliminary stage of data analysis, body image is showing itself to be a key factor in a woman's ability to enjoy, develop and maintain intimate relationships.**

Following on from this is the fact that only 5% of the women felt they look the best they ever have, with only a further 10% slightly agreeing that they look the best they ever have — leaving 85% who do not think they look the best they ever have.

From this we can assume that the vast majority of women who participated in the study feel that they looked their best ever at some point in their past.

What will be interesting to investigate in the future is how many of these women believe that they can look their best ever again in the future? Do they think that their greatest years, in terms of looking and feeling their best, are all in the past?

Congratulations! You're not perfect

It's ridiculous to want to be perfect anyway. But then, everybody's ridiculous sometimes, except perfect people. You know what perfect is? Perfect is not eating or drinking or talking or moving a muscle or making even the teensiest mistake. Perfect is never doing anything wrong — which means never doing anything at all. Perfect is boring! So you're not perfect! Wonderful! Have fun! Eat things that give you bad breath! Trip over your own shoelaces! Laugh! Let somebody else laugh at you!

Perfect people never do any of those things. All they do is sit around and sip weak tea and think about how perfect they are. But they're really not 100% perfect anyway. You should see them when they get the hiccups! Phooey! Who needs 'em? You can drink pickle juice and imitate gorillas and do silly dances and sing stupid songs and wear funny hats and be as imperfect as you please and still be a good person. Good people are hard to find nowadays. And they're a lot more fun than perfect people any day of the week.

STEPHEN MANES,
AUTHOR OF *BE A PERFECT PERSON IN JUST THREE DAYS!*

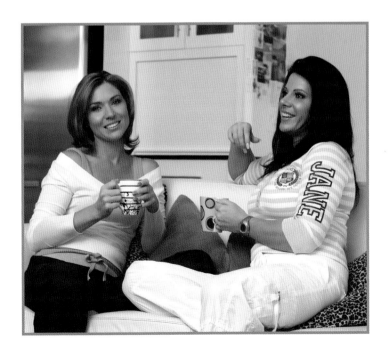

The Psychology of Weight Loss

With clinical psychologist Dr Angela Huntsman

You have to stay in shape. My grandmother, she started walking five miles a day when she was 60. She's 97 today and we don't know where the hell she is.

ELLEN DEGENERES

What's *your* kryptonite?

Our relationship with food is complex. It hasn't always been that way, however – our relationship with food has become more complicated as our options have increased. We make it complex because of the easy choices we now have and the ways in which we emotionally hold ourselves prisoners to not finding truth. The choices we have in our food interfere with much of the simplicity of life. Supermarkets can overwhelm us. How many times have you gone to the supermarket and shopped for what seemed like a large amount of food, yet not actually come home with one complete meal in your shopping bags?

Food is one of those things that seems to have the power to control us. To put it another way: **food taps into a part of** *ourselves* **that we do not seem to have control over.**

Yesterday I stopped by a friend's house to pick up a book she was lending me. She asked what I was doing and I replied, 'I'm writing a piece about our relationship with food.' To which she replied in her beautiful clipped British accent, 'Oh god, don't ask me about MY relationship with food.' And I realised that we all have this 'thing' with food. We always seem to want more. More of something – sweet for some, savoury for others. But there is *something* out there that is our 'kryptonite' … it weakens us and we crumble.

As a psychologist I think that taking apart an issue is more important than working to figure out how it got there in the first place. Why? Well I think that with human beings the 'how things got that way' explanations are either:

a) All in the past

b) Nothing we can change

c) Just 'excuses' waiting to happen.

So when I work with people we start with 'What are we choosing to do *now*?' What do we need to understand about what prevents us choosing exactly what we want right now? There is no tomorrow, there is no yesterday. In the world of absolute reality, there is only NOW. Right now, what do you want? Do you want to eat less? Feel better? Understand why food has power over you? Understanding it will still not give you results. Controlling the hand that feeds you – your own hand – will.

Through the span of human history, whenever food was scarce we went into survival mode. We ate what we found and left it at that. It is when food is plentiful that we start to struggle.

When man foraged and hunted for sustenance, the relationship with food was simple. Man simply ate what he found, when he found it. There was no internal conversation with the self that went like this, 'Hmm, a blueberry bush ... well, I'm not exactly in the mood for blueberries right now. Maybe I'll just keep looking for something I am really craving.' No, actually this is how it went: 'Blueberries, are they edible? Yes!' And eating would take place until either the hunger subsided or the little blueberry bush was picked bare. True hunger has no choices to make. It takes what it finds and consumes it on the spot.

Self-control

Self-control lies behind lots of things we want for our life. Waiting for results is harder in our instant world of today. Instant music, instant photos ... Are you old enough to remember getting photos printed from film? Waiting was required. These instant things in our lives have eroded our sense of self-control. If you don't have to wait for anything you don't really need self-control, do you? Well the plain fact of the matter is – when it comes to our health, nothing gets done without self-control.

Look at your life for evidence of self-control

Are there places where you have masterful self-control? Do you organise your finances beautifully? Do you have orderly closets with clothes all lined up by colour or season? Or a system for keeping track of birthdays? This would equal the place where you are connected to your self-control — a place you have chosen to be important. Okay then. Now take that self-control and apply it to food. We all have self-control that we have access to somewhere. We just need to put it where we need it for the moment — until new habits are formed.

Your body serves a great purpose

Your body is a tool that you use to roam this earth. It was given to you out of the simple miracle of the joining of the egg and sperm that created you. And food is simply the thing that you use to fuel your mind and body. See it as fuel, and not as something to delight yourself with on an as-needed basis. Food can be delightful, beautiful and tasty, but it doesn't *always* need to be those things. Slow it down. Make food simple in your life while you take the time to make other things fabulous. Feed your mind with ideas, get connected to people, care for your home and your heart.

Don't wait for that wake-up call

We don't need to wait until we get a life-threatening illness to get our act together. If the act you need to get together revolves around food, then sit down and start writing, talking and indulging in the thoughts and feelings you have not just about food, but about everything. Food can certainly be a great comfort to us, but if food is your only means to comfort yourself then you have surely sold yourself short. What are other ways you can be good to yourself? A walk around the block for fresh air? A warm aromatic bath? A great book? A tiny amount of time delving into a hobby you love.

Is food really all there is? What are you blocking? Are you a perfectionist? Do you have to hide your problems from yourself so you can look good? Look in control? Well, it is time you joined the human race and gave yourself the grace to be human. You will be a better person to yourself, your husband/partner, your children and friends if you can share the things you struggle with. Chances are when you divulge, others will start to give more of themselves to you. And the support to be had by those around you and the support you can give yourself first is important.

Get happy

The best appetite-suppressant is happiness. We forget about food, we are engaged and interested in things we are doing. A lot of us eat when we are bored. This isn't good – but you know that. Rather than fighting 'boredom eating' as a stand-alone behaviour, why not attack what caused the boredom eating to begin with. Make your life more interesting. Become more engaged and present in everything you do.

When eating is the most fun thing we can think of doing, it is a sad state of affairs. We have all been there and done that, squandering the moments that make up our lives. Is this what you want to remember as you look back on your life? Is this what you want on your gravestone – 'Kinda had an interesting life – but didn't really push the envelope'?

Get real

If you still find that you simply can't control what you eat, then you need to look for runaway trains in your life that you are hiding from, and uncover what the food in your life is blanketing over. We certainly do not need a perfect life in order to eat within healthy limits. But we need to know exactly where we stand in life in terms of marriage, parenting, relationships, home and health.

Nothing and no one is perfect. I don't know anyone with a perfect life. The secret is not trying to reach some ideal standard, but just getting completely clear with where you need to pay attention and do some work and where things are easy and free for you. Then when you worry, you won't sit around and eat – you'll get busy making a difference in those things that are amiss at the moment. This is what we mean by life being a juggling act. And to fall into bed at the end of each day, thoroughly exhausted, and knowing that in everything you did, you did the best you could do that day, is what living a life examined means.

Not everything that can be counted counts,
and not everything that counts can be counted.
ALBERT EINSTEIN

CRASH DIETING

For my son Josh, a yo-yo is one of the best toys ever invented and a source of constant fascination. For the rest of us, however, the word yo-yo is more likely to be associated with dieting, and for some people with years of frustration, pain and anguish.

What causes the yo-yo effect?

Crash diets are linked to the yo-yo effect because of the impact this type of starvation diet has on your body's metabolism. Your metabolism is the rate at which your body burns calories during the course of a day. Your body is incredibly clever in that when it realises it is receiving a very low number of calories each day, it reduces the number of calories required to perform all of its necessary bodily functions. What's more worrying, however, is that your body can maintain this decreased metabolism for a number of months, or even years, after a serious low-calorie diet.

The repercussions for your body of crash-dieting are serious, resulting in short- and long-term health complications that you don't want to experience, including:

Mental health problems

Severe calorie restriction can set you up for the downward spiral into depression. It can also be the starting point leading to eating disorders like anorexia and bulimia. Eating disorders are known to be among the hardest illnesses to treat, and mothers are no less susceptible to developing them than any other group.

Other serious implications of repetitive yo-yo dieting include:
1. Nutritional deficiency
2. Vital organ damage
3. Osteoporosis

Losing weight the healthy way

If you really need to lose weight, it is imperative that you avoid crash diets at all costs. Instead, begin a healthy weight-loss program that focuses on sound nutrition and regular exercise. There is simply no other way to ensure a healthy, long-term love affair with your body.

The positive effect of kindness on the immune system and on the increased production of serotonin in the brain has been proven in research studies. Serotonin is a naturally occurring substance in the body that makes us feel more comfortable, peaceful, and even blissful.

In fact, the role of most antidepressants is to stimulate the production of serotonin chemically, helping to ease depression. Research has shown that a simple act of kindness directed toward another improves the functioning of the immune system and stimulates the production of serotonin in both the recipient of the kindness and the person extending the kindness. Even more amazing is that persons observing the act of kindness have similar beneficial results. Imagine this! Kindness extended, received, or observed beneficially impacts the physical health and feelings of everyone involved!

DR WAYNE DYER

Cravings versus true hunger

With Dr Angela Huntsman

There is hunger for ordinary bread, and there is hunger for love, for kindness, for thoughtfulness; and this is the great poverty that makes people suffer so much.

MOTHER TERESA

Food glorious food

Have you ever been camping? Have you ever noticed that food tastes so good when you are camping? Let's look and see what we have going on here. When we are camping we have relatively little access to prepared food. We don't have cupboards full of food calling out to us or neon signs beckoning us toward fast-food restaurants. No, we are left to be at one with nature. Setting up tents, a place to sleep, somewhere to prep meals and perhaps a good spot to eat. Before we know it, our tummies are growling and with nothing more than a roast onion and a couple of trout cooked in butter we can be in heaven. That is a simple relationship with food. When you are hungry *enough*, the food available (whatever it might be) tastes delicious.

Try this next time you go into the kitchen to eat. Stop at the first thing you find: a can of beans, crackers, leftover pasta ... whatever it is. If none of those things appeal to you, if you are craving something a little yummier, more gooey, perhaps a little sweeter, then turn yourself around and head back out of the kitchen — fast! Take yourself outside and have a stroll in the fresh air. Stop what you were about to do, which was to feed a craving and not an appetite.

Be prepared

What we really need is to have food prepared ahead of time for us to eat. Don't paint yourself into the fast food corner — with low blood sugar, five dollars in your pocket and nothing in your possession to eat. Put a banana, nuts, cheese and crackers into your bag in the morning and when you get hungry enough, they'll taste great.

We are bombarded with weight-loss solutions offering to help us get healthy and fit. There are more products to help us sustain our health than ever before, yet we avoid the simplest things our body asks for: real food, in real amounts, at real intervals.

Things to do differently

Try shopping at the outer walls of the supermarket. You will normally find the dairy, meat, fruit and vegetables there. What about in the middle? All the manufactured food science can create — some with a shelf-life longer than your mortgage, thanks to even more chemicals. Try to avoid these aisles for a month. Just imagine what not having the snack foods handy would do to your chances of success?

Some of us eat badly so we can beat ourselves up. Well, let's be honest, when we are in a bad mood, or anxious or tired, doesn't it just feel like we *deserve* a little treat to help us feel better? Doesn't that little voice then come along, more critical than your own mother-in-law, and start in on you? We all know the drill, it goes something like this: 'Have you no willpower? You'll never make those goals. Now you'll get bigger and you will never look like you used to look and you will be miserable forever if you don't lose weight.'

First of all, losing weight might be associated with being happy, but being thin is no guarantee you will be happy. It's time to start choosing to like yourself, no matter what. Can you give yourself the gift of that which you give to your children and those around you?

The simple truth is that the secret of weight loss is eat less, move more. The shortest chapter in this book.

You have to choose to make this a simple process. You have to choose not to eat when you are emotional. You have to choose not to buy the kind of food that isn't good to have at home. You do not need a food consultant to walk you up and down the aisles reading labels. If it has a label that you don't understand, then don't buy it. Wait until you are really hungry and eat 'clean' food that you can easily understand … fruit and vegetables don't even need a label! This kind of transformation is important.

Keep in mind the fact that your body doesn't gain weight without your consent. You have exactly the kind of body you are feeding. The choice you need to make is in your determination and drive. Do you want it? Do you care? If you don't really want it or care, then give it all a break and go focus your energy on something else for a while. Don't create unnecessary drama in your life — either you are ready to change or not. It's that simple.

If we're not willing to settle for junk living, we certainly shouldn't settle for junk food.

SALLY EDWARDS

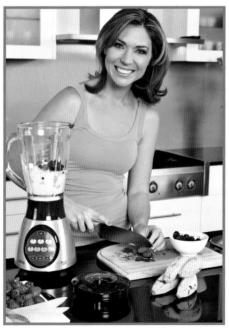

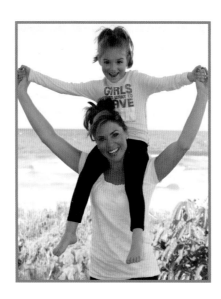

It's all about LOVE

I have found that if you love life,
Life will love you back.

ARTHUR RUBINSTEIN

Louise Hay is the author of *You Can Heal Your Life*, one of the best-selling self-help books ever written. She has a powerful, love-based philosophy, which has not only helped millions of people around the world improve the quality of their life, but also assisted her to completely heal herself of cervical cancer within six months.

Her key messages to us as women include:
- Every thought we think is creating our future
- The point of power is always in the present moment
- Resentment, criticism, and guilt are the most damaging patterns
- We must be willing to begin to learn to love ourselves
- When we really love ourselves, everything in our life works

and most poignantly for us mothers ...
- The bottom line for everyone is, '*I'm not good enough*'.

How comforting to know that we are not alone every time we find ourselves dwelling on the reasons why we are so unworthy of life's abundance? When you think about it, the reason we don't just start living the life we truly want (start that business/ask that man out on a date/put in a request for a raise/demand that we be heard by those in positions of authority … the list is endless) is *always* because of a fear that we are not good enough. (This is usually accompanied by another illogical yet equally immobilising fear, that we will be laughed at and/or rejected.)

Once you understand that 99.9% of people are walking around feeling the same way as you, you can more easily begin to put your insecurities aside and start behaving differently. You won't feel such a need to scrutinise every word you say, every email you send, or over-analyse every conversation throughout each day. You begin, slowly, to get on with the *living* of your life. Which, after all, is what we are really here to do.

When we were children we didn't think, 'When I grow up, half my day will be spent worrying about what others think of me and the other half will be spent wondering whether or not I am good enough to even be here.' No, we thought about becoming a dancer, a doctor, a movie star or a policewoman … we assumed we could fit all of those careers into the course of our life, and the idea of being worthy or good enough to do any of them was about as preposterous as wanting to eat vegetables at a birthday party!

So what happened along the way? Did motherhood erode our sense of self-worth to such an extent, or did this begin a long time ago and motherhood merely became the final act in a Shakespearean tragedy created purely in our minds?

Take a moment now to reflect on the love that exists in your life today – most importantly, your ability to give and receive self-love each day.

The greatest gift you will ever receive is the gift of loving and believing in yourself.
Guard that gift with your life. It is the only thing that will ever truly be yours.
TIFFANY LOREN ROWE

Post-natal depression

CASE STUDY
Christine, mum of two

This is what post-natal depression feels like ...

Take your worst hangover and prolong it for months. Erase humour from your personality. Add self-loathing, and the belief that you're a waste of people's time. Experience things that give you pleasure as if they are unpleasant chores.

Your thoughts are rigid and you can't organise yourself to do something as simple as chopping an onion. You're desperate to rest but sleep doesn't come, or is snatched cruelly from you when everyone else is breathing rhythmically. Weld to your nerves a jangling anxiety as you rush on full-speed adrenalin towards the catastrophes that you know await you.

Cry uncontrollably and wish you could be beamed up into space rather than go through your life. Wear a mask of reality, so no one knows your misery, and use every ounce of energy to pretend you're okay — or just a bit tired. Wonder what the hell is wrong with you. Now look after a baby and a toddler. That's post-natal depresssion.

EXTRACT FROM *NEXT* MAGAZINE, NEW ZEALAND

After *You Sexy Mother* came out, I received thousands of emails from mums, many of whom shared their stories of experiencing and coping with post-natal depression. Although I was never diagnosed with PND, I feel very connected with this debilitating illness because to me there is such a fine line between experiencing a challenging time as a new mum but surviving it, and crossing over to a place where you feel completely out of control and disconnected. I am passionate about highlighting post-natal depression, and sharing the stories of women who have come out the other side and are willing to share the strategies that worked for them.

Post-natal depression is treatable, and there are things that others can do to make an enormous difference to a mum who is affected by it. We all need to be vigilant, as it can affect any new mum and there is no way of knowing who will and won't be affected. By offering as much support as possible to any new mums in your life, you will be doing your bit to make it that much easier for them to get through those first few critical months, when sleep deprivation and a sense of isolation can be overwhelming.

I was asked to speak at a post-natal depression support group here in my community on the Sunshine Coast in Australia soon after *You Sexy Mother* was released. I met some of the most remarkable, competent, high-achieving and beautiful women at that group, and together we laughed and cried our way through an afternoon where we were all able to lift the veil of motherhood and be true to our own feelings of self-doubt and insecurity. From that moment onwards I found myself becoming passionate about doing all I could to raise awareness of PND. I now work closely with an amazing psychologist, Lisa Lindley, who devotes many unpaid hours each week to helping those mums on the Coast who are feeling overwhelmed and undersupported. Courses are run for eight weeks, and during that time I have watched so many women transform and blossom into not only the women they used to be, but so much more.

We recently took the PND group one step further and have initiated an exciting project called M.A.D. — 'Mothers' Adventure Days' — where we take to the mountains, the river and the sea to pursue activities that push us out of our comfort zones and remind us what it is to be a woman who is fully alive, not just a mother responsible for the needs and wants of those around us.

We have been abseiling down sheer rock faces, and both my kids have been out at sea paddle-boarding with us mums. We have kayaking and windsurfing lined up for the near future, and who knows where this simple yet powerful idea will take us? I sent information about our local M.A.D. initiative out to my *You Sexy Mother* community around the globe, and we had so many eager mums get in contact, wanting to know how they could start similar groups in their hometowns.

I love the idea that we are now talking about and actively working together to destigmatise the label 'post-natal depression'. It is becoming something that has hope attached to it, rather than simply fear and shame. We are showing that as well as medication, there are options in terms of physical activity and social connectivity that can greatly help mums who are suffering. If we can create fun, supportive environments for mothers who are affected by PND, where they can spend time together and support one another, then we are moving in the right direction.

If there are two things connected to motherhood that deserve to be held up to the light and discussed in a respectful and honest way in the 21st century, they are post-natal depression and pelvic floor dysfunction.

We are making good progress thanks to wonderful organisations such as Panda and Beyond Blue in Australia and similar wonderful initiatives in other countries, and with the help of passionate and knowledgeable people such as Mary O'Dwyer, who conducts pelvic floor seminars and workshops around the world.

If you think you might be experiencing depression of any kind, I urge you to reach out to someone and ask for help. It might be your doctor or maybe a friend – if you can bring yourself to share your true feelings with just one other person, I can assure you it will be the start of something more positive in your life. You might prefer a friend or family member to talk to a doctor on your behalf and find out what the next step should be. Just having someone else you trust make the call and book an appointment with your doctor can make it so much easier. If they can go with you and hold your hand while someone else looks after your children, then that is even better. There is so much power in reaching out to someone and telling them how you are really feeling … it truly is the beginning of the healing process.

Some of the warning signs to look out for in yourself and others include:
· a prolonged period of feeling low or 'blue'
· reduced interest in activities – especially those you used to really enjoy
· tiredness and sleep disturbances
· changes in your appetite
· negative thoughts and feelings
· feeling overwhelmed
· anxiety
· irritability and angry outbursts
· the inability to laugh and enjoy yourself.

Actual percentages vary, but in general it is thought that 15% of mothers experience post-natal depression. It can affect anyone, and there is no typical group of women who are more likely to experience PND.

This book is dedicated to the simple idea of feeling good in your physical skin. Not looking like a bikini model, not living up to some perfect ideal clothing size – just feeling good inside and out. Post-natal depression makes achieving that goal a challenge for any mum, and makes working out or in some cases even getting out of bed very difficult. Let's work together to support and encourage one another to take baby steps towards total well-being.

If you would like to learn how you can get involved in some *You Sexy Mother* events as well as specific PND initiatives, please visit the website and sign up to the community. This is a vital and very engaged group of amazing women, who all share a desire to live a full and vibrant life as mums.

What lies behind us and what lies before us are tiny matters
compared to what lies within us.
RALPH WALDO EMERSON

THE INTERNATIONAL MOTHERHOOD STUDY
Expectations

The International Motherhood Study allowed us to investigate whether or not a woman's expectations of motherhood were matched by the reality. Are we prepared for what awaits us when we become mothers ... can we ever be prepared for motherhood?

The results were highly variable. Whilst 21% of mums strongly agreed that their experience of motherhood had not been what they expected, 22% disagreed with this statement, implying that in fact motherhood was as they expected. The remaining 57% were fairly evenly spread across the continuum, indicating that we all come to motherhood with varying expectations. For some of us, motherhood takes us completely by surprise, while others seem to sail through effortlessly by comparison.

Interestingly, expectations were shown to have a statistically significant effect on a mother's mental and emotional health. Those mums who felt that their expectations had been met were in a much healthier place in terms of their depression, anxiety and stress scores (as measured against the internationally recognised 'DAS' – Depression, Anxiety and Stress measurement tool). Those mums who felt their expectations had not been met, reported significantly higher levels of depression, anxiety and stress.

We can see that expectations prior to motherhood are an important factor in determining the emotional well-being of a mother post-baby. This indicates that encouraging realistic expectations prior to motherhood could be a vital tool in assisting women during this major life transition.

CASE STUDY
Meg, mum of two

Going it alone – Meg chooses exercise over antidepressants and develops her own health and fitness program to transform her life.

Were you always a fit and active person?

I wouldn't say I've *always* been fit and active. Since my early twenties I've gone through spurts of interest in the form of gym memberships, but the spurt usually lasted six to eight months at best.

How would you describe your fitness during pregnancy?

A friend and I would swim for 40 minutes once or twice a week. During my second pregnancy I was lucky enough to discover a local community centre which offered a great range of facilities, making it easy and enticing for me to exercise. There is a well-managed crèche, a gym, swimming pool and café.

Can you tell me what happened during and after your most recent pregnancy?

I wish I could say I enjoyed being pregnant, but sadly I didn't. My hormones ran rife right from the beginning. My skin looked like a spotty hormonal teenager's and my cup size grew from D to well past H! This meant I had a lot of trouble breastfeeding. I had been told by doctors in advance that I might not be able to feed, so I thought I was well equipped to cope with whatever the outcome was. I certainly was not prepared for the hormones that follow childbirth, which instruct every cell in your body that as a female you were designed to breastfeed come what may!

My family live in another state and I just craved that unconditional support and understanding, without the advice that is so often given with the best of intentions, whether wanted or not.

When my second son was three months old, we decided to sell our house. All the pressure that comes with presenting a spotless package for weeks on end were slowly bringing me undone. Not to mention the move at the end of it all! I'm a bit of a control freak too, and I wanted to be seen as being able to cope with all aspects — because after all, I chose to be a mother, and now I'll do my damnedest to do it perfectly. I didn't want to let on that I was struggling. I didn't want to be the one being talked about.

At what point did you realise that you were in a bad place emotionally, spiritually or physically?

When my second son was about six months old I remember feeling like I was riding an emotional rollercoaster. Occasions that should be filled with joy left me smiling on the outside but feeling hollow inside. I felt overwhelmed and out of control, in every respect. A simple trip to the supermarket, friends dropping by unannounced, a pile of washing could undo me at any moment. I didn't even feel I had the enthusiasm to talk on the phone with friends, it all felt too hard. Not only was I feeling emotionally overwhelmed, physically deflated and mentally too tired to manage much more than the basics, but I realised that by giving myself wholeheartedly to motherhood and domesticity I had lost myself. I was taking my role as stay-at-home mum too seriously. It was all I lived, thought about and talked about, and it was not healthy for my sons, my husband and most of all myself.

Did you seek help or visit a doctor?

During a doctor's visit for my son, she asked me how I was doing. At that, I burst into tears. I felt safe enough to share with her all the emotions that had been building up for months.

What was your response to her advice and recommendations?

The advice provided was that she thought I was suffering from depression. The recommendations were varied, from being prescribed antidepressants, taking up exercise and making time for myself to reading about forms of relaxation and meditation. I wholeheartedly understand the need for some people to take antidepressants for myriads of reasons, but I felt I needed to explore the other options suggested first. I felt I needed to give myself a chance at regaining some sense of 'me' again with a more natural approach. So herein started my own personal challenge

What was the turning point that made you decide to prioritise your health and fitness?

I didn't want to feel like this any more — I basically had no other choice but to rediscover myself and start enjoying this blessed life. I wanted to wake up each morning and feel like it was going to be a good day.

Where did you start/who helped show you the way?

I must have been starting to send out positive vibes because a number of stars aligned for me and I started to feel some good energy coming my way. I drew strength and confidence from the encouraging words in the book *You Sexy Mother*. In particular those relating to making time to exercise, and where there is a will there is a way. I really felt like Jodie was talking to ME! I could relate to every word and I felt like I had someone on my team. Couple this with the support of my husband, who was prepared to do whatever he could to help with getting me back on track, and I was on my way. This started off with him taking over with the boys when he got home from work so I could go for a walk. Only two or three kilometres at first, but I found I was really starting to enjoy this exercise business. There's a lot to be said for fresh air and time to clear one's head. I started to set a few simple goals for myself and within a few months I was running 5 km and looking forward to it. I even entered a local fun run and exceeded my expectations.

What does your nutrition and training look like each week now?

I've built my two gym workouts into our weekly routine so that each week there is dedicated time for me. My local community centre offers a wonderful crèche which the boys love, and this is extremely important to me. If it didn't work for the family, it couldn't work for me. Because I have worked my gym time into our schedule each week, it means there are no excuses, no reasons to back out. I've always been a foodie and really into cooking. So not only is it important that I nourish our family with fresh healthy food, but I make sure I have fun with it each week. This is my creative outlet and a chance for some of that relaxation my doctor was referring to.

What keeps you motivated?

I think there are a number of factors that have to work together to keep you motivated. For me, I really wanted things to change and this thought is powerful enough to keep me focused. A significant positive side effect of this is the physical condition I am enjoying. To see and feel the changes, and to be receiving compliments along the way, keeps me coming back for more. The satisfaction of achieving my own set challenges each week/month is so rewarding. Pushing through and succeeding gives me a huge buzz. I also find that the uninterrupted time for me to think and dream ensures I stay focused on the wider picture. It gives me a chance to reassess and reprioritise.

What have been the best bonuses of leading an active life as a mum?

I feel so much stronger, both physically and mentally. I also love that natural high I get from the endorphins surging through my body, and also the feeling of success that I get from achieving each little challenge I set for myself. I feel like I have taken charge of my sense of self again. I do also feel that I am a good role model for my boys. To be able to put myself out there and encourage a healthy approach where I take control and lead by example is very important to me.

Sexy from the inside out

You should spend your money on some nice lingerie.
Big cotton pants, that just doesn't work. You have to feel sexy!
HEIDI KLUM

Sexy, alluring, desirable – whatever you call it, that need to be desired and indeed loved never really goes away. But as most mothers will attest, it does seem to fade into the background (or rather we do!) if we don't work at it.

The basic premise of the *You Sexy Mother* philosophy is that sexy is more of a feeling than an outward image. Like being in control of your life, sexy is a state that comes from within – a projection of confidence and self-assuredness that attracts others to us like a magnet.

Underneath a woman's clothing, who's to know what colour and style of underwear she is wearing? We might not be able to see it, but success leaves clues, and it's no different when it comes to what we put closest to our skin.

If you are yet to experience the difference between wearing a gorgeous set of matching lace underwear versus mismatched grey cottons, then you are in for the ride of your life. Get into your wardrobe now and fish out all those gorgeous silky items you have been saving for that special occasion or for that moment in time when your body/hair/relationship/house/kids are perfect.

Get them out, put them on and experience the glorious sensation of feeling that you are worthy of them in this moment – just the way you are.

I repeat: just the way you are!

Realise you have choices and can decide at any moment to do things differently. You can literally become sexy from the inside out, because being sexy has very little to do with panting and purring in stilettos and a great deal to do with valuing and respecting yourself as the magnificent, emerging woman you are – one who is worthy in this moment, in this body, with this amount of money in the bank. You are worthy simply because you are you.

Don't stop there, by the way – while you are delving into the back of your underwear drawer, why not take a look in the back of your bathroom cabinet? I'll bet there are all sorts of goodies waiting patiently for their perfect moment in time too — expensive eye creams, decadent body lotions and luxurious, sweet-smelling handcreams all eagerly awaiting that special day when you will deem it acceptable to open and use them. Who are you kidding? We all know that day will never come and eventually they will either end up as last-minute gifts for unsuspecting friends or they will expire along with your dwindling sense of self-worth.

Why not decide that today and indeed the rest of your life is special enough and reason enough to celebrate! Go on, be brave … open them up and squirt them ceremoniously over your lingerie-clad body. Embrace the feeling of decadence, and declare to anyone who will listen (yes, even the mirror will suffice), 'I am worthy of using and enjoying the best that life has to offer!'

Much like happiness, I believe we are about as sexy as we make up our minds to be!
Choose well and enjoy all that life has to offer.
EXTRACT FROM *YOU SEXY MOTHER — THE JOURNAL*

Sex appeal is fifty percent what you've got and fifty percent what people think you've got.
SOPHIA LOREN

This is an actual extract from a sex education school textbook for girls, printed in the early 1960s in the UK, and explains why the world was much happier and more peaceful then …

When retiring to the bedroom, prepare yourself for bed as promptly as possible. Whilst feminine hygiene is of the utmost importance, your tired husband does not want to queue for the bathroom, as he would have to do for his train. But remember to look your best when going to bed. Try to achieve a look that is welcoming without being obvious. If you need to apply face-cream or hair-rollers, wait until he is asleep as this can be shocking to a man last thing at night. When it comes to the possibility of intimate relations with your husband, it is important to remember your marriage vows and in particular your commitment to obey him.

If he feels that he needs to sleep immediately then so be it. In all things be led by your husband's wishes; do not pressure him in any way to stimulate intimacy. Should your husband suggest congress, then agree humbly all the while being mindful that a man's satisfaction is more important than a woman's. When he reaches his moment of fulfilment, a small moan from yourself is encouraging to him and quite sufficient to indicate any enjoyment that you may have had.

Should your husband suggest any of the more unusual practices, be obedient and uncomplaining but register any reluctance by remaining silent. It is likely that your husband will then fall promptly asleep, so adjust your clothing, freshen up and apply your night-time face and hair care products.

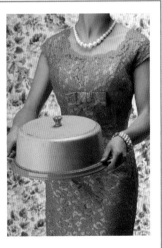

You may then set the alarm so that you can arise shortly before him in the morning. This will enable you to have his morning cup of tea ready when he awakes.

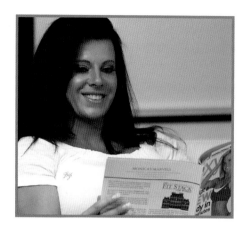

Final words from Kelli

Most people never run far enough on their first wind to find out they've got a second. Give your dreams all you've got and you'll be amazed at the energy that comes out of you.

WILLIAM JAMES

This collaboration with Jodie has been an amazing journey for both of us. Jodie came to me a long time ago with a very clear goal to learn simple, effective strategies that would help her look and feel the way she wanted to, for the rest of her life. Not a quick-fix or miracle cure, but a realistic and proven formula for creating a strong, vital, *sexy* body.

I have wanted to share my extensive knowledge on this subject with women the world over for many years now. I have dedicated my life to learning how to balance health and fitness with the at-times overwhelming demands of being a mum, wife, sister and friend. It has been such an honour to share my experience and expertise with you, and I have complete confidence in your ability to use this information to go out and experience life in a whole new way.

You don't have to wonder how those wonder-women do it any more — thinking there is some secret code or secret society of mums that you will never belong to. This lifestyle plan is for everyone and WORKS for everyone. I have trained with every kind of woman imaginable, from those looking to lose a lot of weight, to those looking to gain curves and increase energy. Without fail, everyone who applied the simple principles you now have, and found within themselves a sincere desire to succeed, changed their lives forever. Some of them even went on to compete and win figure competitions — something they had never even considered before.

What I want to emphasise is that no matter where you are now and how far away your end goal may appear — you have everything you need right here in your hands! If you would like to contact me about anything you have read in this book or would like to take your training to the next level, please feel free to visit my website www.keljohnson.com.

I wish you every success and hope that you return to this book whenever you feel the need to renew your confidence and restore your faith that what we have told you works!

Finally, my number-one secret of success is this ...

Set a goal, take action, go for it!

WITH LOVE, KELLI x

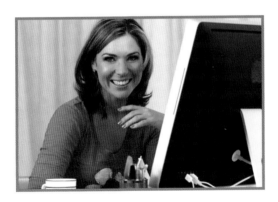

Goodbye from Jodie

One of my favourite quotes, which popped out at me during the writing of this book, is this one from the model Twiggy:

I was always insecure about my looks. I never, ever loved what I looked like.
Now, with the benefit of hindsight, I can see that I was different ...
What I have learned is that every woman has something special and unique.

When you realise that even supermodels and so-called 'perfect' women (yes, that includes Halle Berry!) have self-doubts and worry about their bodies, you start to see the futility of wasting too much energy analysing your every bump and dimple.

For me the quest is, and always has been, about energy. Getting it, keeping it and using it to design my life, the way I want it. If you've got energy and a few dimples here and there, who cares? If you've got the body of Kate Moss but no energy to run around having fun with the kids, what's the point?

Try to find a happy balance within all of this. Try to connect with what really lights you up inside, and learn to laugh a lot more about the trials along the way than you cry over your apparent failures. We can't exist in an airbrushed world of perfection, and most of us wouldn't want to.

Sexy isn't about the state of our lingerie drawer — it's about the way we carry ourselves, the energy we radiate toward others. It's about charisma, self-love and choosing to look at our smile in the mirror instead of at our stretch marks. The secret is focus — the ability to focus on the things that truly matter and to ignore the rest. The hardest part is learning how to differentiate between the two.

As always, I encourage you to visit me at www.yousexymother.com.au to continue your journey and to share with others the way in which your life has been transformed.

Thank you for allowing me, through these pages, into your life, heart and home.

The firsts go away — first love, first baby, first kiss.
You have to create new ones.
SARAH JESSICA PARKER

Defining moments

Two roads diverged in a yellow wood and I,
I took the one less travelled by
And that has made all the difference.

ROBERT FROST

I vividly recall the day when my *You Sexy Mother* career and life might just as easily have become another 'coulda/shoulda been' in my life. Just another missed opportunity that I could have packed away in that suitcase of great ideas and big dreams that until this moment had lain hiding under my bed where no one else could share my pain and sadness.

Just one week earlier I had sat around the dining-room table at my friend's house, excitedly sharing my dream of writing a mother's inspirational handbook with a friend of hers who was a freelance editor. This woman had kindly agreed to look over the manuscript and give me some guidance before I sent it off to various publishers. I remember feeling so happy that I was finally on my way, and courageously handed the manuscript over before spending a rather tense week waiting to reunite and receive the feedback.

Now here we were again, my friend and I enjoying some polite chit-chat as the editor entered the house. We sat down, and I admit to being somewhat worried as I noticed the strange, almost expressionless look on her face as her eyes darted everywhere about the room except at me. Finally I wearied of the small talk and blurted out, 'So, did you get a chance to look over my manuscript? What did you think?'

'To be honest,' she started hesitantly, 'I just don't know who you think is going to buy this book. You talk about making motherhood fun and turning "chores into blessings", and having "date nights" with your husband. I have never ironed a thing and I can't remember the last time my husband and I had a night out together. To be honest, I just don't think anyone is going to *buy* this book!'

Taking a deep breath, and with a calm inner strength that I didn't even know I possessed at that time, I looked her in the eye and said, 'I didn't ask you if you *liked* my book, I asked you if it was grammatically good enough to send out to publishers next week.'

'Oh yes, grammatically it's fine,' she told me.

'Great,' I continued, 'here's your money ... thank you for your time.'

Here was the perfect opportunity for me to admit defeat and listen to the 'experience and wisdom' of someone who was already in the publishing industry. What did I know about all this?

Luckily, something deep within me spoke up loud and clear. So she didn't like the book — so what? She wasn't my target mum, and no book could possibly appeal to every mother. I was writing a book for mums who wanted more out of their motherhood journey — mothers who wanted to live an *exceptional* life, not just go through the motions. I made up my mind that she was wrong and I was right, and by the time I got round to telling this story to large groups of mums, I was speaking at the Sheraton Hotel in Noosa, Australia.

I had just returned from a publicity tour of New Zealand where my book *You Sexy Mother — a life-changing approach to motherhood* had just hit the best-seller list. Australia's Channel 9 were at the hotel filming me for a segment that was going to air that night across the nation. In the audience were representatives from one of Australia's leading professional speakers' bureaus, who within a week of the event had booked me for four major speaking engagements throughout Australia. Just weeks before I had launched the International Motherhood Study across Australia and New Zealand and I was in the process of finalising parallel studies to be released in the US and UK.

I shared with the women in the room my gratitude at being mentored by New Zealand's 'Veuve Clicquot Business Woman of the Year', Annah Stretton, who had recently agreed to help me take my vision of empowering mothers globally to the next level. Then I told of how I had been speaking alongside New Zealand's Minister for Women's Affairs, Pansy Wong, and how in one surreal moment after the next had found myself accepting her kind offer to put a signed copy of my book on the Prime Minister's desk the next day. 'He needs to read this,' were her words.

It was a hugely gratifying moment — sharing this story of one woman's attempt to end my dream and vision before it had even begun with an audience who in many cases were welling up with emotion as my own voice faded in and out as I tried to relive this fragile moment of time in my life.

There had been other times in the past when I had let the voices of others dictate my life and my idea of what I could and couldn't achieve — friends, teachers, parents, well-meaning yet small-minded colleagues ... luckily for me, this time I wasn't going to let it happen again. Instead I decided to use this editor's feedback as leverage or motivation — if only to show her that she was wrong, and that perhaps she didn't know as much as she thought she did. I was going to make sure I saw this dream to the very end — no one individual would be able to pour cold water on my vision this time. It would take an army of dream-snatchers to stop or even slow me down ... and the rest, as they say, is history.

I hope this book and my story act as a catalyst in your life. I want you to know that I didn't have a million dollars in the bank, or a team of supporters cheering me on from the sidelines. I was you — I was a normal woman, mum, wife, sister, friend who wanted more.

More fun. More excitement. More fulfilment. More joy. More of the good stuff. Reading this book could be the defining moment in your life, if you let it.

Take the first step in faith. You don't have to see the whole staircase, just take the first step.
MARTIN LUTHER KING JR

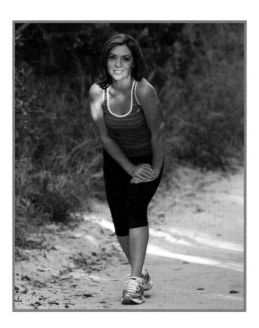

Body Bible Tool Box

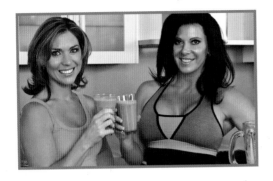

Nutritional programs

1. Five-day detox program
2. Nutritional option 1
3. Nutritional option 2
4. Nutritional option 3
5. Mini-meal options
6. Shopping list

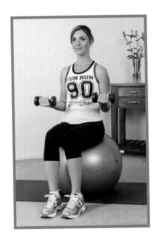

Training programs

1. Home-based program
2. Gym-based program
3. Travel program
4. Baby-buggy program
5. Core/abdominals specific program
6. Stretching routine

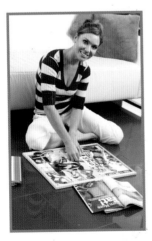

Success tools

1. Vision board
2. Vivid goal-setting
3. Self-audit
4. Training planner
5. Training journal
6. Success roadmap
7. Create a new story

Nutritional programs

PLEASE NOTE

As we are all starting out from a different place in terms of our nutritional and/or weight-loss goals, the following nutritional plans represent an *example* of what your new diet might include. They are designed to show you how you can put the nutritional principles you have learnt about in this book into practice in your day-to-day life.

If you have any medical conditions that need to be considered, please make sure you see your doctor before making any significant changes to your diet. If you are unsure about any aspect of these nutritional plans, please seek the advice of a qualified dietician or your doctor.

Key points to remember:

1. You can eat more or less of the foods included in the meal plans depending on your level of physical activity and your personal health and fitness goals.

2. You need to drink 8+ glasses of water a day (more if you are exercising).

3. If you are vegetarian or vegan, please substitute appropriate protein sources where necessary.

4. The consumption of supplements and protein powders is optional, depending on your personal preferences, unique goals and current state of health.

1. Five-day detox program

Depending on the state of your current diet, embarking on a detox program can sometimes be a bumpy road with many highs and lows initially. However, the feeling of clarity you get and the wonderful end result are so worth it, so hang in there and stick to your plan! You may wish to buddy up with a friend so you are able to support each other when you are feeling low – most likely during the first few days. Get out for walks together and share your experiences along the way.

This might be a good time to get out your journal and start writing – detoxing can bring up a lot of 'stuff', including emotional issues such as unresolved or unpleasant experiences. Take it slowly and realise there is a powerful transformation process taking place.

It is important that you reintroduce foods slowly once you complete the five days. Your body will be much more sensitive to foods – especially fast food and highly processed foods. Be aware of how your body reacts to the different foods as you reintroduce them.

Most importantly, be kind to yourself. Do not overload yourself with extra work or commitments during this time. Try to get to bed early and pamper yourself a little bit more than normal. Remember that you are trying to create healthy habits for the future – not further stress your body with rapid, extreme and unsustainable changes.

Key points to remember on the detox plan

1. Within reason, you can eat more or less of the foods included in the detox program. Listen to your body and your own hunger cues to guide you.
2. Remember to eat every three hours from your first meal!
3. You need to drink plenty of water – aim for 2-3 litres of water throughout each day.
4. Keep your exercise moderate – 30-40 minutes of brisk walking, swimming, yoga or pilates would be perfect.
5. Start the day with a glass of water with a squeeze of lemon or lime. This will get your digestive juices going.
6. If you are vegetarian or vegan, remember to substitute appropriate protein sources where necessary.

Five-day detox program – daily meal plan

Meal 1   2 cups of mixed fruit salad
(include bananas, grapes, mango, blueberries, strawberries,
oranges and kiwifruit)

   +

Multivitamin tablet (optional)
Omega-3 tablets (optional)

Meal 2   2 cups of mixed fruit salad

Meal 3   1 serve tuna (in spring water)
Large green salad (may include green olives, capers,
lemon juice)
Small serve of feta or cottage cheese
Steamed brown rice

  or

1 serve chicken or turkey breast
Large mixed salad
Steamed sweet potato

Meal 4   Protein shake (30-g serve of protein powder mixed with water)
3 rice cakes with reduced-sugar jam

Meal 5   1 serve lean steak, chicken or turkey breast meat
2 cups steamed vegetables

  or

1 serve fresh fish
2 cups steamed vegetables

Meal 6   Cup of herb tea
Apple or piece of fruit

* Season food with fresh herbs, lemon juice, Mexican seasoning, balsamic vinegar,
olives and capers.

2. Nutritional plan 1

Meal 1   Bowl of rolled oats (sweeten with honey and sultanas)
Protein shake (30-g serve of protein powder mixed with water)

+

Multivitamin tablet (optional)
Omega-3 tablets (optional)

Meal 2   2-3 rice cakes with:
• 2 tbsp cottage cheese (approx)
• 120 g sliced turkey, chicken or ham
• sliced tomato

Meal 3   1 serve tuna in spring water (or lite tuna option)
1 serve sweet potato
1 cup of steamed vegetables or mixed salad
(season with lemon juice, fresh herbs, olives, capers and
balsamic vinegar as desired)

or

Pita bread pizza – top one wholemeal pita bread with tomato-paste,
tuna and olives (or any combination of your favourite
healthy toppings)
Serve with mixed salad

Meal 4   Jodie's Super Smoothie (see Recipe section)
or

1 of Kelli's Choc-Peanut Protein Balls (see Recipe section)

Meal 5   1 serve lean steak, chicken or turkey breast
Large serve of steamed vegetables or mixed salad
(season with lemon juice, fresh herbs, olives, capers and
balsamic vinegar as desired)

or

1 serve salmon or white fish
Large serve of steamed vegetables or mixed salad
(season with lemon juice, fresh herbs, olives, capers and
balsamic vinegar as desired)

Meal 6   1 piece of fruit
Cup of herb tea

3. Nutritional plan 2

Meal 1   1–2 slices of rye/wholegrain toast spread with avocado
Egg omelette with baby spinach, tomato and cumin

    +

                Multivitamin tablet (optional)
Omega-3 tablets (optional)

Meal 2   Protein shake (30-g serve of protein powder mixed with water)
1 banana or apple, nectarine, peach or pear
Cup of green tea

      or

                Fresh or frozen berries and yogurt smoothie with a small scoop
of protein powder, water and ice.

Meal 3   1 serve sliced chicken, turkey or ham
1 rice bread (mountain bread) or rye/wholegrain roll
Mixed salad
Cottage cheese or natural yogurt

Meal 4   2–3 rice cakes with peanut butter

      or

                Small serve mixed raw nuts and sultanas

Meal 5   1 serve lean beef or chicken mince (see Recipe section)
Wrap in cos lettuce leaf parcels
Serve with large mixed salad (season with lemon juice, fresh
herbs, olives, capers and balsamic vinegar as desired)

Meal 6   Reduced-sugar jelly
Cup of herb tea

4. Nutritional plan 3

Meal 1   Bowl of natural muesli, Special K or Sultana Bran
(or other high-fibre cereal)
Protein shake (30-g serve of protein powder mixed with water)

+

Multivitamin tablet (optional)
Omega-3 tablets (optional)

Meal 2   1 serve natural (or low-fat flavoured) yogurt
1 banana

or

Smoothie
Mix yogurt, banana, water and ice with 1 tsp LSA (ground linseed, sunflower seeds and almonds) in a blender

Meal 3   1 serve chicken, turkey or tuna
1 rice or rye bread wrap
Green salad with avocado

Meal 4   Protein shake (30-g serve protein powder mixed with water)
Handful of raw mixed nuts

or

1 of Kelli's Choc-Peanut Protein Balls (see Recipe section)

Meal 5   Chicken and vegetable kebabs
(try cherry tomatoes, mushrooms and zucchini)
Place cubed raw chicken breast with mixed vegetable cubes on a skewer and barbecue or grill to perfection
Serve with extra vegetables or side salad

Meal 6   Baked apple with a drizzle of honey and cinnamon

5. Mini-meal options

Use the examples below as a starting point for creating nutritious, high-energy snack options to help you feel full throughout the day.

There are endless options available when it comes to creating healthy meal choices to fill up on at regular intervals throughout the day. The hardest part can often be trying to incorporate some form of protein into most of your meals. Keep in mind that protein is essential for your muscles — without enough protein you cannot create (or maintain) enough muscle to keep your metabolism kicking along and burning up the calories you take in each day. The more muscle you have, the more your body burns calories even when you are sedentary — it's really important therefore to maintain and build your muscle, whilst encouraging your body to burn fat for energy.

Select from the options below during the day and try to include some form of protein with at least four of your five to six meals. You will see protein powder incorporated into several of the options, as this is often a convenient and easy way to ensure your body gets enough protein throughout the day.

- Rice or corn cakes topped with a variety of fillings:
    tomato, cottage cheese and chives
    avocado and a squeeze of lemon
    small spread of cream cheese or cottage cheese, seasoned with fresh herbs
    peanut butter
    sugar-free/reduced-sugar jam
- Mix 1 tub of yogurt with 1 scoop protein powder and put on top of a bowl of fruit salad
- Pita bread pizza — top 1 wholemeal pita bread with tomato-paste, tuna and olives (or any combination of your favourite healthy toppings)
- 1/2 cup mixed natural nuts (almonds, cashews and hazelnuts)
- Chocolate and peanut protein balls (see Recipe section)
- Fresh veggie sticks (carrot, celery, capsicum, green beans) with avocado dip (1/2 mashed avocado with lemon juice)
- Scrambled eggs with baby spinach
- Smoked salmon rolls filled with chopped parsley and sprouts or rocket salad
- Chicken and vegetable kebabs — place cubed raw chicken breast with mixed vegetable cubes (try cherry tomatoes, mushrooms and zucchini) on a skewer and barbecue or grill to perfection

- Devilled eggs — cut hard-boiled eggs in half lengthways. Remove yolks and set whites aside. Combine cottage cheese, light mayonnaise, mustard and yolks in a bowl and mash with a fork until well blended. Quantities will vary according to the number of eggs being used. Add chopped chives if desired. Refill whites, using about 1 tablespoon yolk mixture for each egg half.
- Banana, yogurt and LSA (ground linseed, sunflower seeds and almonds) smoothie. Blend with water and ice
- Fresh or frozen berry and yogurt smoothie with a small scoop of protein powder, water and ice
- Baked peaches with cinnamon and a dollop of mascarpone cheese (a special treat!)
- Baked apple with a drizzle of honey and cinnamon
- Fruit and nut mix

Recipes

It was never the intention of this book to offer specific recipes and dietary plans to be strictly adhered to. The main aim is to provide you with key nutritional principles so you can adapt and enjoy recipes from the many wonderful cookbooks available and learn to eat out and make good food choices regardless of where you are.

The following recipes are just a few suggestions from within this book to get you started, but we encourage you to start adapting the recipes you already enjoy as you introduce more fruits, vegetables, 'good' carbohydrates and lean protein to your diet.

TASTY CHICKEN DELIGHTS

Take 500 g of sliced chicken breast and marinate it briefly with chopped fresh garlic, a whole squeezed lemon, chopped basil and coriander, along with some salt and pepper and a drizzle of good oil (macadamia or coconut oil are great).

Cook in a non-stick pan until ready. These flavoursome chicken pieces can be put into a rice bread wrap with salad for lunch along with a drizzle of natural yogurt, or served with vegetables or salad for a tasty dinner.

HOMEMADE HEALTHY MINCE PATTIES
(the kids will love these too!)

Combine 500 g lean mince with tomato paste and seasoning (you can use any chilli or satay-style seasoning you like depending on how hot you like it). Mix to a good consistency then form patties and fry them in a non-stick pan. These patties are tasty for the whole family and are perfect to put into a wrap along with your favourite salad ingredients.

Another option is to take the cooked mincemeat (don't roll into patties) and add finely diced cucumber, red pepper and fresh herbs before wrapping it all up in a large lettuce leaf.

CHICKEN MINCE PATTIES

Combine 500 g chicken mince with Greek yogurt (approx 125 g), toasted pine nuts, fresh chopped coriander and some salt/pepper. This mixture can be formed into patties (roll into a ball and cook in a non-stick fry pan) then added to a wrap with salad and peanut butter for extra protein and flavour – delicious!

KELLI'S CHOC-PEANUT PROTEIN BALLS

  I cup rolled oats
  I cup chocolate protein powder
  2 tbsp low-fat chocolate drinking powder
  200 g peanut butter
  I/4 cup honey
  I/2 cup chopped natural peanuts, almonds or cashews

Place rolled oats, protein powder and drinking chocolate in a bowl and mix with a hand blender or food processor until the oats are powdery. Stir in the honey, peanut butter and nuts. When mixed thoroughly, roll into balls and refrigerate.

Eat and enjoy – perfect for your post-workout fix of carbohydrates, fat and protein!

JODIE'S SUPER SMOOTHIE

banana

honey

cinnamon

peanut butter

LSA (linseeds, sunflower seeds and almonds)

1 serve (30 g) vanilla protein powder (optional)

yogurt

water and ice

Blend it all up for a nutritious (and delicious) mini-meal any time of day. Yum!

6. Shopping list

This is what I like to call Kelli's 'No excuses' shopping list!

You should be able to make healthy, nutritious meals that are quick and easy if you always keep the following ingredients stored in your fridge or cupboard.

Use this list as a starting point for your new focus on healthy, high-energy eating, and add your own list of items that you find and love as you go.

The fresh stuff

- Any fresh herbs that you like (especially coriander and basil)
- Sweet potato
- Capsicum (red, yellow and green)
- Any and all vegetables — especially green! (Lettuce, spinach, rocket, zucchini, broccoli, Brussels sprouts …)
- Berries (full of antioxidants)
- All fruit — including bananas, peaches, pears, pawpaw, mango and nectarines
- Tomatoes
- Avocado
- Lemons

Protein sources

- Eggs, egg whites
- Lean chicken mince, chicken tenderloins and chicken breast fillets
- Turkey breast
- Lean beef mince
- Eye fillet steak (or any lean cut of beef)
- Fresh fish (all kinds)

Starchy carbs (best eaten early in the day or just after exercise)

- Wholegrain bread
- Brown rice
- Sweet potato
- Wholegrain pasta
- Rye bread
- Rice bread
- Rice or corn cakes
- Wholegrain cereals – natural muesli
- Oats
- Corn
- Peas
- Pumpkin

A little bit of dairy

- Natural yogurt
- Trim milk
- Cream cheese
- Cottage cheese
- Lite cheese

In the cupboard

- Dry seasonings
- Tinned corn
- Tinned tuna
- Tinned pineapple pieces
- Sundried tomatoes
- Olives
- Capers
- Almonds – plus mixed raw nuts
- Peanut butter
- Reduced-sugar jam
- Honey
- Protein powder
- Reduced-sugar jelly
- Sultanas
- LSA (ground linseed, sunflower seeds and almonds)

Just for taste

- Mexican spice
- Lemon pepper
- Soy sauce (or 'Bragg's all natural, liquid aminos' – a soy-protein, soy-sauce substitute, available at health food stores)
- Curry powder
- Thai spice
- Tomato paste
- Indian spice
- Balsamic vinegar

My shopping list …

Training programs

1. Home-based program
2. Gym-based program
3. Travel program
4. Baby-buggy program
5. Core/abdominals workout
6. Stretching routine

Intensity

As you get stronger you can increase the intensity of the programs by increasing the weights where appropriate (making sure you don't sacrifice technique) and by completing the exercises in less time. You can decrease the rest periods in between but you do need to have *some* rest/recovery time to ensure you do not put unnecessary strain on your body or injure yourself. This is particularly important for women who have pelvic floor issues that need to be considered.

Key points to remember

Try to aim for 3 x resistance training sessions each week (30 minutes using weights or a physio-band at home or at the gym) along with 3-4 cardio sessions (working at a moderate to vigorous intensity for 30+ minutes). You can simplify things by combining your cardio workout and resistance training exercises where possible – this way you reduce the number of sessions required each week to start seeing results. Make sure you give yourself rest and recovery days during the week too.

1. Try to do exercises in front of a mirror to ensure you use the correct technique throughout.
2. Maintain the correct posture by growing tall through the crown.
3. To help ensure correct technique, begin by using light weights and build up slowly.
4. Start with 10-12 repetitions x 1-2 sets, gradually building up to 20 repetitions x 3 sets.
5. Remember to breathe – always breathe out as you lift or push a weight.

Pelvic floor reminder

While exercising be aware of your pelvic floor. If it pushes down or out as you exercise, stop, rest, then choose an easier exercise option. All women benefit from learning the correct pelvic floor/core muscle action before they begin an exercise program.

Before beginning each exercise remember to draw up and hold your pelvic floor muscles as this switches on the important abdominal and core muscles (transversus abdominis and deep spinal multifidus). Many women have been incorrectly taught to simply pull in and narrow their waist but this trains our abdominals incorrectly. You must *start* by drawing up your core muscles from underneath your body.

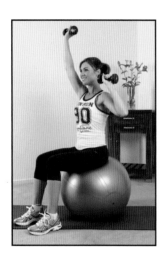

1. Home-based program

Equipment required
· Fitball
· Set of dumb-bells (2 kg, 3 kg or 5 kg)

1. Seated alternate shoulder press

1. Sit on the Fitball with your feet flat on the floor. Shoulders are back and down.
2. Bend your elbows and place your hands in front of your shoulders with the palms facing forward.
3. Raise the dumb-bell above your head in a straight line, then return to start position. Repeat on the other side.

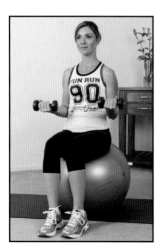

2. Bicep curls

1. You may sit on the Fitball (with your feet flat on the floor) or stand for this exercise.
2. Place both arms down by your sides, holding the dumb-bells with the palms of your hands facing up.
3. Curl the dumb-bells upwards and towards your body either alternately or together.

3. Tricep kickbacks

1. Kneel on the floor, resting on one hand. Keep your spine straight (neutral position).
2. Hold the dumb-bell with your palm facing inward. Keep your upper arm tucked closely into your side and your elbow up.
3. Curl the dumb-bell towards the front of your shoulder/armpit, then push the dumb-bell backwards until your arm is straight and near your hips.

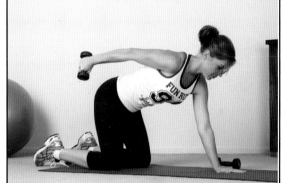

4. Return to the start position and repeat for one full set before using the other arm.

4. Chest press

1. Lie down with your back resting on the Fitball.
2. Roll forward until your upper back, shoulders, neck and head are supported on the Fitball.
3. With your feet slightly wider than your shoulder width, raise your hips until you are parallel with the floor. Hold your glutes tight and switch on your pelvic floor and core muscles to maintain this position.

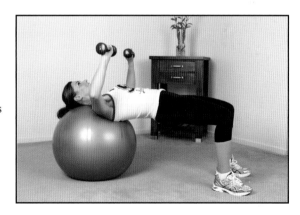

4. Place the dumb-bells in front of your shoulders and together press them to the ceiling so the dumb-bells almost meet in the middle at the top.

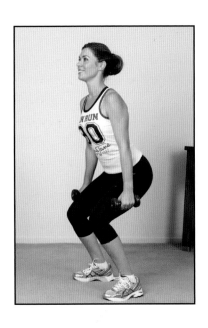

5. Squats

1. Stand with feet slightly wider than shoulder width apart and keep your heels on the ground throughout the entire movement.
2. Place your arms by your sides while in the standing position, then bend your knees.
3. Remember to keep your chest up and stick your bottom out behind you when you squat.
4. Always push up through your heels. If you find your heels are coming off the ground, widen your stance until such time as you are more conditioned to this exercise.

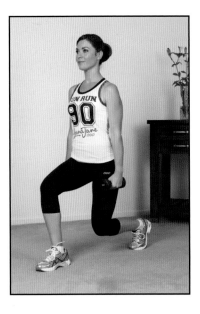

6. Lunges

1. Place one foot forward and one foot behind you and keep the heel of the front foot on the ground throughout the entire movement.
2. Lower your bottom straight down towards the floor, allowing the heel of the back foot to come off the ground.
3. Then push your body upward again with your weight through the heel of the front foot.
4. Make sure your feet are wide enough so as not to place strain on the knees.

7. Core/abdominals

Select from the exercises in the Core/abdominals workout (page 217).

2. Gym-based program

Ensure you enlist the help of a qualified fitness professional when embarking on any training program at a gym. You need to feel confident that you can use all the equipment safely and that you are using the right weight to ensure proper technique and reduce any chance of injury.

It is always a good idea to review your program and technique with a staff member at regular intervals (every 4-6 weeks).

1. Seated lat pulldowns

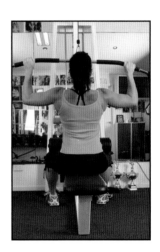

1. Sit with your knees under the roll pads.
2. Hold the wide grip bar, just outside of the bend (on the bar).
3. Stay tall and lean your upper body slightly back (keeping this position).
4. Pull the bar downwards to the centre of your chest, using your back muscles (lats), then control the weight as the bar moves up to the starting position again.
5. Repeat slowly, breathing out as you pull the bar down.

2. Seated row

1. Sit on the bench with your feet on the foot rest and your knees slightly bent.
2. Pull the handle towards your rib cage and squeeze the muscles between your shoulder blades together.
3. Allow the bar to return to the starting position
4. Maintain a tall sitting posture and pivot through the hips (do not allow your back to hunch over in the forward position).
5. Maintain smooth repetitive movements and breathe out as you pull the handle to your chest.

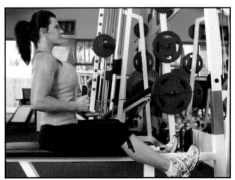

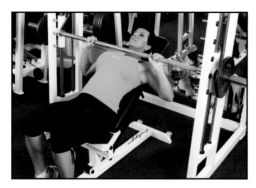

3. Chest press (incline)

1. With the adjustable bench positioned at 45 degrees, sit on the bench, resting back.
2. Bend your elbows and place your hands in front of your shoulders with the palms facing forward.
3. Press the bar toward the ceiling then lower it back down to your chest.
4. Always maintain pelvic floor, core and abdominal control.

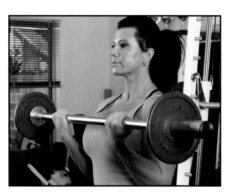

4. Barbell bicep curls

1. Stand with your arms by your sides, holding the barbell with your palms facing upwards.
2. Keep your upper arms close to your body.
3. Curl the barbell up towards your shoulders then slowly lower to the starting position, bending at the elbows only. Repeat.

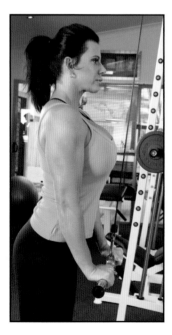

5. Tricep pushdowns

1. Stand at the tricep machine (or cable machine) and hold the straight bar.
2. Your elbows should be bent, with your hands in slightly closer than shoulder width.
3. Your upper arms are pressed in against your body.
4. Push the bar downwards and squeeze the back of your arm (tricep).
5. Allow the bar to move upwards again, keeping your upper arm against your body so your hands do not come up past your chest.
6. Stay tall and breathe out on the downward movement.

6. Leg press

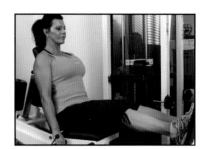

1. Sit with your feet placed in the middle of the platform, slightly closer than shoulder width apart (always keeping your heels on the platform).
2. Push upwards, being careful not to lock your knees out at the top of the movement.
3. If your hips rotate and your glutes move forward you have gone too far with this movement.
4. Control the weight carefully as it comes back down.
5. Remember to breathe out as you push through your heels with pelvic floor, core and abdominal tension.
6. If your pelvic floor pushes down, then stop, relax and remove some weight before restarting the exercise.

7. Leg curls

1. Lie face-down on the bench with your feet under the roll pads and your knees just over the end of the bench.
2. Hold the handles and curl your heels back towards your glutes and down again.
3. Continue smooth repetitive movements.

8. Shoulder press

1. Sit on the upright bench with your back fully supported and feet flat on the floor.
2. Hold your hands in front of your shoulders with the palms facing forward.
3. Press the dumb-bells upwards, almost meeting in the middle at the top of the movement, and back down to starting position.

9. Core/abdominals

Select from exercises in the Core/abdominals workout (page 217).

3. Travel program

Equipment required
- Exercise band/physio-band

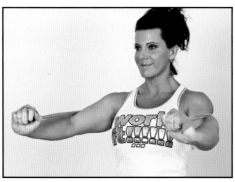

I. Chest press

1. Standing tall, hold both ends of the exercise band and place it behind your back just under shoulder height. (Adjust the band length for resistance.)
2. Holding the handles on the band, press alternate or both hands forwards in front of your chest (maintaining chest height).
3. Using a controlled motion, allow the band to return to the start position, then repeat.

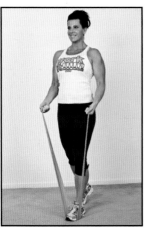

2. Bicep curls

1. Stand with one or both feet on the centre of the exercise band.
2. Hold the handles with your palms facing forward and curl your hands up towards your shoulders.
3. Slowly lower back down and repeat.

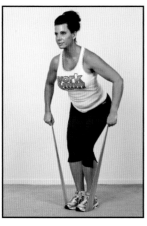

3. Back rows

1. Stand with one foot (or both feet for more resistance) on the centre of the band.
2. Bend and lean slightly forward, palms facing forwards.
3. Draw back both elbows, squeezing your back muscles together.
4. Control the band as your hands move forward, and repeat.

4. Squats

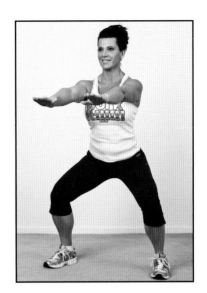

1. Stand with your feet slightly wider than shoulder width apart and keep your heels on the ground throughout the entire movement.
2. Place your arms by your sides while in the standing position, then bend your knees, raising your arms up and in front of you while in the bent-knee position.
3. Remember to keep your chest up and stick your bottom out behind you when you squat.
4. Always push up through your heels. If you find your heels are coming off the ground, widen your stance until such time as you are more conditioned to this exercise.

5. Lunges

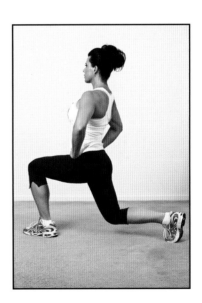

1. Place one foot forward and one foot behind you, and keep the heel of the front foot on the ground throughout the entire movement.
2. Lower your bottom straight down towards the floor, allowing the heel of the back foot to come off the ground.
3. Then push your body upward again with your weight through the heel of the front foot.
4. Make sure your feet are wide enough that you don't put strain on the knees.

6. Core/abdominals

Select from exercises in the Core/abdominals workout (page 217).

4. Baby-buggy program

Equipment required
- Baby buggy
- Park bench

1. Start with a brisk walk while pushing the buggy.
2. Aim for a minimum of 30 minutes and extend the time as your fitness increases.
3. Whilst pushing the buggy try some walking lunges.
4. When the buggy is stationary try squatting.
5. If you are near a park you can use a bench to do some tricep dips and step ups.
6. Select appropriate exercises from the ab/core workout that follows if time (and baby!) allows.

Lunges

1. Place one foot forward and one foot behind you, and keep the heel of the front foot on the ground throughout the entire movement.
2. Lower your bottom straight down towards the ground, allowing the heel of the back foot to come off the ground.
3. Then push your body upward again with your weight through the heel of the front foot.
4. Make sure your feet are wide enough so you don't place strain on the knees.

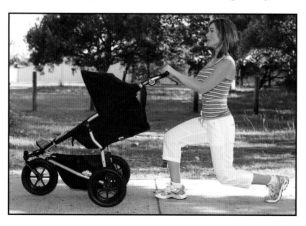

Squats

1. Stand with your feet slightly wider than shoulder width apart and keep your heels on the ground throughout the entire movement.

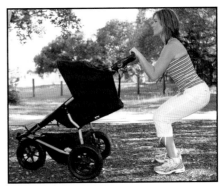

2. Place your arms by your sides while in the standing position, then bend your knees, raising your arms up and in front of you while in the bent-knee position. Alternatively, you can keep your hands on the buggy throughout the exercise.

3. Remember to keep your chest up and stick your bottom out behind you when you squat.

4. Always push up through your heels. If you find your heels are coming off the ground, widen your stance until such time as you are more conditioned to this exercise.

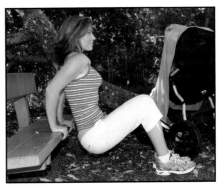

Tricep dips

1. Sit on the bench and place both hands down, holding the edge (hands facing forwards).

2. Place both feet flat on the ground out in front of you.

3. Slide your bottom off the bench and lower yourself towards the ground.

4. Push yourself up with your arms.

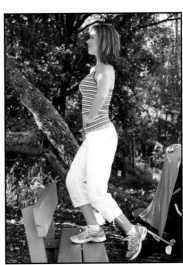

Step ups

1. Placing one foot flat on the centre of the bench, lift your body up and back down again.

2. Alternate legs for every step up.

5. Core/abdominals workout

Equipment required
- Fitball
- Medicine ball (optional)

It is very important that you select abdominal exercises that are appropriate for your level of fitness and personal circumstances. If you have recently had a baby or have any pelvic floor concerns whatsoever, only perform the first three pelvic floor approved exercises. You can progress to the more challenging exercises as your fitness improves and your pelvic floor muscles strengthen.

Key points to remember

1. Start with one set of 10-12 reps and slowly progress to 3 sets of 20 reps.
2. Before beginning each exercise remember to draw up and hold your pelvic floor muscles.
3. Many women have been incorrectly taught to simply pull in and narrow their waist but this trains our abdominals incorrectly. You must *start* by drawing up your core muscles from underneath your body.

Beginner/pelvic floor approved exercises

1. Superwoman

1. Kneel with your hands under your shoulders and knees under your hips.

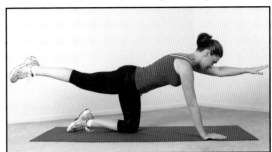

2. Imagine you are balancing a stick across your lower back, and keep it balanced as you stretch one arm out overhead with the opposite leg behind. Hold and breathe for 10, then repeat with the other leg.
3. Repeat 5 times each side.

2. Leg holds

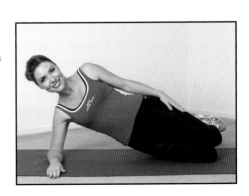

1. Lie on your back, with legs raised and bent. Your hands are behind your head, supporting your neck.
2. Breathe out as you engage your pelvic floor muscles and lift your head and shoulders slightly off the floor. Hold for 5-10 seconds.
3. Remember to maintain a small gap between your lower back and the floor (avoid flattening).
4. Repeat 10 times slowly.

3. Side bridge

1. Lie on your side with both knees bent to a 45-degree angle and your feet together.
2. Prop yourself up on your forearm and push up through your elbow.
3. Lift your hips up off the ground so your body is level; hold for 5, then lower with control. Repeat 5-10 times each side.

Intermediate/pelvic floor approved exercises

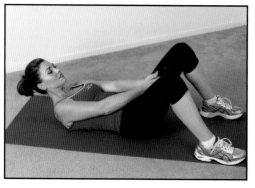

1. Wide leg glide

1. Lie on your back, both knees bent, feet on the floor. Both the knees and the feet are wide apart.
2. Maintain a small space under your lower back as you bring your head and shoulders forward.
3. Both arms are straight and slide through your open legs.
4. Hold and breathe for 5–10 seconds, relax, then repeat slowly 5–10 times for 1–2 sets.

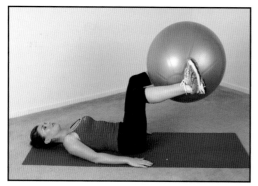

2. Fitball lift

1. Lie on your back and place a Fitball between your feet.
2. Maintain a small curve in your lower back as you bend and keep both knees facing up towards the ceiling.
3. Slowly lift and lower the ball only from your knees (keep the small curve in the lower back).
4. Repeat 10 times slowly for 1–2 sets.

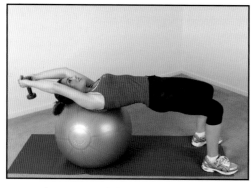

3. Fitball hold

1. Hold onto a 2-kg weight. Lie down on the Fitball so it is supporting you under your neck and shoulders.
2. Your feet are shoulder-width apart and your bottom is lifted, so your body becomes like a table top.
3. With straight arms, lift the weight from above your tummy back over your head, returning to the tummy position.
4. Repeat the action without any ball movement 10 times slowly, for 1–2 sets.

Kelli's advanced ab/core exercises

1. Fitball crunches

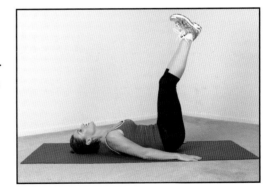

1. Sit on the Fitball and roll slightly forward until the middle of your back and shoulders are supported.
2. Place the palms of your hands together and under your chin. Tuck your chin down on your hands.
3. Draw up your pelvic floor muscles and tighten your abdominals from right down just above your hip bones.
4. Once you can feel them tight, move your upper body in a curling motion towards your hips.
5. Try not to let the Fitball move underneath you. If it is rolling around, you are not using your abdominals correctly.

2. Hip raises

1. Lie flat on the floor with your feet together and arms down by your side.
2. Bend your knees and lift both feet up until they are above your hips.
3. Point your toes and lift your pelvis off the floor towards the ceiling and back down again, keeping your feet off the ground.
4. Continue this small movement, making sure you draw up and hold your pelvic floor muscles throughout the exercise.

3. Bicycles

1. Lie on your back on the floor with your fingertips gently touching your ears.
2. Lift both feet off the floor until they make a right angle behind your knees.

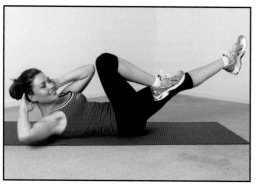

3. Raise your shoulders slightly off the floor.
4. Bring your opposite elbow and knee together to meet in the middle of your body, while straightening the other leg out but keeping your foot off the ground (like pedalling a bicycle).
5. Repeat on the other side.

4. Alternate medicine ball crunches

1. Lie down on your back with your legs and feet on the floor.
2. Your hand should be above your head, holding a medicine ball.

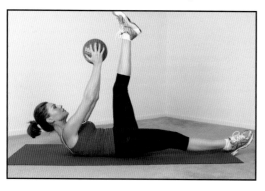

3. Bring the medicine ball up over your head towards the centre of your body while at the same time raising one leg straight up to meet the medicine ball in the middle of your body.
4. Lower the medicine ball back behind your head at the same time as you lower your leg to the ground.
5. Repeat using the other leg.

6. Stretching routine

It is very important that you perform a general warm-up (at least five minutes of aerobic activity such as brisk walking, jogging, jumping rope, or any other activity that will get your blood pumping) before you stretch. It is never a good idea to attempt to stretch before your muscles are warm as this can lead to injury.

Key points to remember

1. Hold each stretch for 20-30 seconds and repeat 2-3 times.
2. Breathe throughout the stretches.
3. Start slowly and add stretch as your muscles relax.
4. Always ensure you perform slow, smooth stretches. Never bounce.

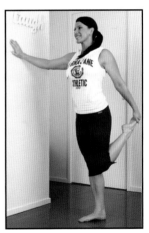

1. Quad stretch

1. Stand and hold onto a support for balance.
2. Hold one of your ankles and pull it up to your bottom, allowing your quad muscle to stretch.
3. Swap to the other side and repeat.

2. Hamstring stretch

1. Sit on the ground with your legs straight out in front of you.
2. Reach forward with both hands and try to touch your toes.
3. This stretch can also be done standing up.

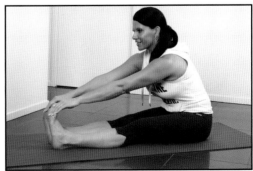

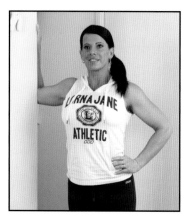

3. Chest stretch

1. Stand in front of a doorway and place your forearms on either side of the doorway with the elbows at shoulder height.
2. Gently lean forward into the doorway until you feel a slight stretch.
3. Rest and repeat.

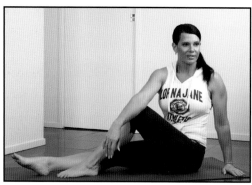

4. Seated back stretch

1. Sit on the floor with both feet out in front of you.
2. Bend your right leg so your foot is in line with your left knee.
3. Stretch your left arm across and behind your right knee so your left elbow is resting on your right knee, keeping your right hand on the floor for support.
4. Gently push your knee and elbow together to provide a gentle stretch.
5. Repeat on the other side.

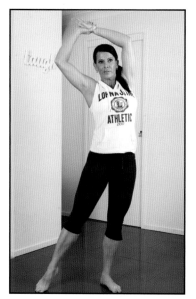

5. Shoulder stretch

1. Stand up with your hands above your head.
2. Clasp one wrist and pull gently to the side of the hand that is holding the wrist.
3. Feel a good stretch down the side of your body, then swap sides.

Success tools

1. Vision board

Create a compelling vision for *your* future ...

If you don't know where you are going, any road will take you there — so the saying goes. Today, grab all the resources you can find, such as magazines and glossy advertising brochures (consider printing out pictures from the Internet if it helps). Using the inspiration that you have found through reading this book, look for pictures and words that resonate with where you want to go in life. Look for anything that moves you in some way or provides a sense of excitement and inspiration for your future.

Select words that encapsulate the feelings and experiences you are seeking — such as 'strong', 'energy', 'vitality' or 'well-being'. Then overlay these words on a board (which can be any size you choose) with pictures that reinforce the main themes of how you see your life in the future.

Don't get too hung up about how you are going to achieve all this, or whether the pictures you have selected are 'realistic' enough. For now just cut and paste without holding back, trusting that if you want something enough, you will find a way to achieve it.

Below is an example of how your vision board *could* look (yes, it's mine!).

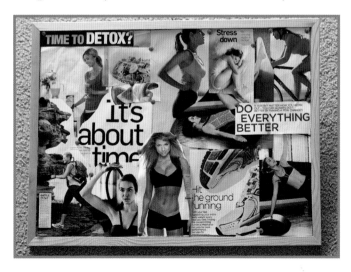

2. Vivid goal-setting

Use the diagram below to help you create specific and emotionally charged goals that will take your life forward in a positive way. For full details on how to do this, refer back to page 147.

Get clear and get excited – that's when you will start to see the results show up in your life

Champion goal	Emotional connection

Inspirational image/representation

3. Self-audit

Self-audit action steps

· Use this self-audit page as a guide.
· On a piece of paper write down all your strengths and weaknesses that you can think of.
· Write down opportunities based on strategies to counteract or improve your areas of weakness. You may have several for each.
· Put your strategies into place and tick them off as they are successfully executed.

For full details on using the self-audit tool refer back to page 145.

Strengths

Weaknesses

Opportunities / strategies

4. Training planner

As with any really useful planning tool, I advise you to be realistic about using this training planner. It is an *ideal* week planner, not a realistic (I can do this 100% every week) kind of tool. Life is simply not designed for that kind of rigid, 'I won' or 'I lost' mentality. We need to plan for success, but build flexibility into any tool.

By looking at the weekly planner that follows, you will be able to decide (perhaps on the Sunday before each new week) what you can realistically commit to over the following seven days. It will give you an opportunity to at least assess whether you are best to work towards a before-breakfast, morning, afternoon or evening training session, and what that activity might be — training at the gym, running around the block or kicking a ball at the park, for example.

Use it to *help* you, not as a tool to beat yourself up with when you don't meet your plan 100%. Be easy on yourself, and set realistic targets with plenty of variety built into your week to help keep motivation high.

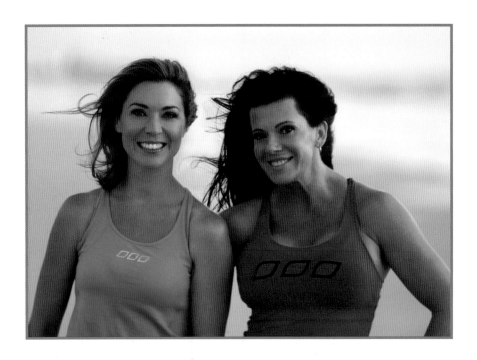

Session	MON	TUE	WED	THUR	FRI	SAT	SUN
Before breakfast			✔		✔		
Morning						✔	
Lunchtime							
Afternoon				✔			
Evening	✔						
Proposed activity: (e.g. running/ gym/swimming)	Gym class		Power walk	Gym class	Run	Yoga	

5. Training journal

This is a simple option to allow you to review your progress and revisit your successes along the way. By checking in daily and weekly to assess the degree to which you are following the nutritional and training guidelines, you give yourself a far greater chance of long-term success.

Put Y in the Nutrition box if you followed the nutritional guidelines.
Put Y in the Training box if you exercised for a minimum of 30 minutes.
Put Y in the Water box if you drank the recommended minimum of 8+ glasses of water.

Be sure to enter your energy level each day, along with the number of hours you slept.

Write down any additional comments that would be good to look back over as you continue to review and revise your program while moving toward your goals.

Additional comments may include information such as:
· Supplements you are taking
· Relaxation or complementary activity — meditation, yoga or sports massage
· Problems you are facing relative to your training goals
· Strategies you discover to assist you with your goals
· Support you received to help you achieve your goals
· Unexpected benefits experienced, such as feeling less anxious or more tolerant of family members
· Compliments received

Training Journal

Week no.

Date:

	MON	TUE	WED	THUR	FRI	SAT	SUN
Nutrition Y/N							
Training Y/N							
Water **(8+ glasses)** Y/N							
Energy level? **1–5** **(low to high)**							
No. of **hours' sleep?**							
Additional **comments:**							

6. Success roadmap

Build your bridge, step by step, from where you are to where you want to be.

I hope you can see from the example below how powerful it is to break down your goals into bite-sized chunks. No matter how lofty or indeed intimidating your goal might seem, anything is possible when you approach it this way. This example is based on one in the *You Sexy Mother* 'Ten-day turnaround plan'.

Create a strong, healthy body

First decide what level of fitness, kind of body or energy level you are aiming for — be as specific as you can. Ten steps is usually a good number to consider when you break your goals down in this way.

1. Commit to working on your goal for five 30-minute sessions per week (minimum).
2. Organise the necessary support people to ensure you can follow through with your commitment.
3. Devise a training routine to achieve your goal (enlist the help of a professional at your local gym if necessary).
4. Keep a training journal to help you on your way.
5. Talk to as many people as you can who are already achieving results in this area.
6. Read as much as you can relating to nutrition and training.
7. Get progress reports by way of gym assessments or fitness tests you carry out periodically. Use these to motivate yourself towards further success.
8. After a period of four to six weeks look over your original plan and the results it has produced — decide to carry on as you are, or adapt your plan/timetable/eating habits etc. to ensure your future success.
9. Be persistent. Keep revising your plan until you reach the results you are after.
10. Celebrate success along the way!

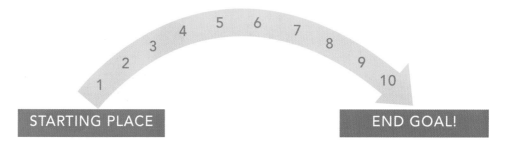

7. Create a new story

Esther and Jerry Hicks, the authors of *Law of Attraction* and numerous other international best-sellers, encourage us to consider looking at the 'stories' we continually tell others about our lives. They argue that by repeatedly saying that we are 'no good with food' or that we 'don't have what it takes' to exercise successfully, we hold ourselves back from ever realising our deepest desires.

We need to stop telling the same old story about how our life didn't go to plan, or how we can't get the body we really want because of some excuse or another built up over years of prolonged story-telling. We each need to rewrite the story of our life and start telling this new revised version to anyone who will listen. Tell yourself at least every night before bed!

By taking an honest look at your 'old' story and really considering how it has limited your life up to this point, you will find all the motivation you need to rewrite the future exactly as you would like it to be.

Use the examples below as a guide to writing or typing up your old and new stories. Commit to reading your new, improved story aloud every night before you go to sleep. Watch as things start to change in relation to what you are now allowing yourself to believe to be true for you.

Be mindful of times when you start retelling your old story to others — this will only sabotage your success and is no longer necessary. If you can't say anything positive to begin with, don't say anything at all. Once you repeat your story every night for a couple of weeks, you will find yourself wanting to share it with others, because it will be coming to life before your very eyes and people will be asking you what your secret is!

An example of your old story ...

I've never been able to control what I eat. Every time I lose weight, I seem to put it back on again and end up feeling stupid. I don't like the gym — I don't know what I'm doing there and everyone else looks so fit already; I just don't belong. My mum said she always struggled with her body after having kids, so I guess I've just inherited this body shape from her. I would like to get leaner and more toned but I really don't want to eat carrot and celery sticks for the rest of my life, so I think I'll just stick to wearing my baggy clothes and hope for a miracle!

An example of your 'new' story ...

I now understand how powerful it is to combine fresh, healthy food and daily exercise. I know that my body is capable of adapting and changing in truly phenomenal ways, and I am confident that if I do all I can each day to make healthier choices I can transform my body into whatever I want. My mind is a powerful force in helping me succeed, so I focus on my goal of looking lean, toned and vibrant and look at the images each day on my vision board to help inspire me. I am determined to follow the success principles from the Body Bible and do something active each day to boost my metabolism. I now eat healthy food regularly throughout the day and allow myself the occasional treat to keep things 'real'.

My clothes are starting to feel looser and I enjoy the feeling of being able to go into my wardrobe and put on anything I want each day. My body is becoming my friend as I take better care of it and it responds by giving me more energy to do all that I want in life. I love feeling in control of my moods and being able to make good choices each day. I do everything I can to become a strong, healthy role model for my kids. I feel so proud of myself and I love the way my body looks and feels.

You can write your new story any way you like — just use the example above as a guide and remember to write your story in the present tense as if it is already happening. That way you can start to experience (in your mind) what it will feel like to succeed and have the body you desire. The next step will be seeing it happen, and that is such a wonderful process!

WHAT'S *YOUR* STORY?

Behind every book is a story — a series of events culminating in the creation of an idea powerful enough to inspire the author to write.

Behind every life is a story — a story of hope, like a silent dream-weaver, influencing the decisions we make to ensure that we become whatever our hearts call us to be.

Motherhood can test all this, as at every moment, on any given day, we are torn between pursuing our own longings and desires and putting the needs and wants of those who depend on us at the forefront. How then do we manage the impossible — following our dreams and obtaining everything we ever hoped for from this life, and being that perfect mother, wife, sister, daughter and friend?

When I started writing this book, I too was confronted by that same contradiction in my thoughts. In the previous few years many wonderful events had taken place.

Yet when my then two-year-old son Josh was diagnosed with coeliac disease, my world came crashing down around me. Everything became incredibly unimportant unless it directly related to improving his health and rebuilding my family unit to full strength.

There is certainly nothing like a health crisis to help you refocus and reprioritise — especially when it affects your children.

That said, I re-emerged from a teary haze, and marathon-like sessions with doctors and dieticians, with a newfound resolve to use this diagnosis as an opportunity to rebuild my life anew. I was already pretty happy with the strategies I had been employing to allow me to become that 'sexy mother' who prioritises self-care and her own passions — integrating them reasonably well alongside a happy, healthy, family life. Yet I felt a calling to go deeper, to uncover more profound areas for transformation as a mum — I wanted to explore the concept of 'living in the magic of life' without the aids of nannies, house-cleaners, a dozen PAs and suchlike. I wanted to access the energy source within, so I could do all that was really meaningful to me, and do it with vitality and enthusiasm.

I have experienced something profound and life-changing as a result of that exploration, and I invite you to embark on a journey like this too — take a trip to a place where motherhood as a concept knows no limits, where sex doesn't end once children arrive, where life gets better one day after the next and where your energy begins to soar to levels you hadn't even experienced in your carefree single days.

My son Josh is now back to full health and I myself have transformed both physically and mentally after learning the fundamental principles of well-being.

This is my gift to you — a decoded, step-by-step guide to reinventing yourself as a mother that is easy to understand and implement. Some amazing women (both famous and not so well known, yet all equally adorable!) have shared their secrets too — so you can fast-track your journey towards achieving the body and life you always wanted.

I hope you have enjoyed the powerful messages this book contains — what it offers is priceless, and so are you.

More inspirational reading

Jim Collins, *Good to Great* (William Collins, 2001).

Louise Hay, *You Can Heal Your Life* (Hay House, 2008).

Esther and Jerry Hicks, *Law of Attraction* (Hay House, 2006).

Stephen Manes, *Be a Perfect Person in Just Three Days!* (Yearling, 1996).

Mary O'Dwyer, *Hold It Sister* (Redsok, 2010).

Joyce Walsleben, *A Woman's Guide to Sleep* (Three Rivers Press, 2001).

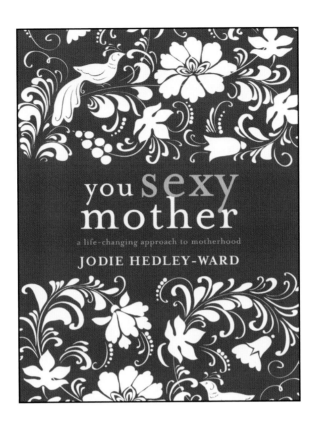

You Sexy Mother **redefines what it means to be a mum today — one who is sexy, vibrant, healthy, happy and engaged in a life that has meaning and value.**

It invites you to look at your role as mother in new and empowering ways, and encourages you to gain more from the experience of motherhood. The author documents her own journey through her personal diary entries, but also incorporates inspirational stories of transformation from other women she has met.

Of special value is the Ten-Day Turnaround Plan — a fast-track programme designed to create explosive positive change and set you on the path to leading the life you truly want and deserve!

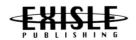

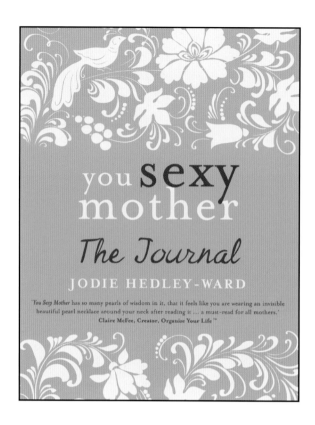

You Sexy Mother — The Journal **is the interactive companion to Jodie Hedley-Ward's best-selling book,** *You Sexy Mother.*

It continues the author's quest to empower women to view motherhood as a catalyst for creating their best life — allowing them to take control and live an authentic motherhood experience.

In the *YSM Journal*, the author offers fresh insights and the wisdom of many great writers. Especially valuable are the 'Reflection Questions', encouraging you to find the right balance in your own life so it is more rewarding, more enjoyable, more sexy. This book also includes the inspirational Ten-Day Turnaround Plan.

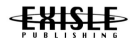

NOTES

NOTES

NOTES

NOTES